Feeding Your Baby

Day by Day

✳ *From first tastes to family meals* ✳

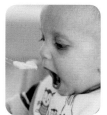 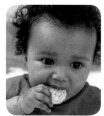 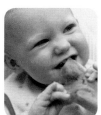 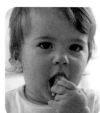

FIONA WILCOCK

LONDON NEW YORK MUNICH MELBOURNE DELHI

DK UK
Senior Editor Claire Cross
Designer Harriet Yeomans
Project Editor Elizabeth Yeates
Senior Pre-Production Producer Andy Hilliard
Senior Producer Oliver Jeffreys
Studio photography Ian O'Leary
Additional photography Andy Crawford
Managing Art Editor Christine Keilty
Publishing Manager Anna Davidson
Art Director Jane Bull

DK INDIA
Editor K Nungshithoibi Singha
Senior Editor Charis Bhagianathan
Senior Art Editor Ivy Roy
Art Editors Zuarin Thoidingjam, Aparajita Barai
Assistant Art Editor Tanya Mehrotra
DTP Designer Sitish Gaur

DISCLAIMER

Every effort has been made to ensure that the information contained in this book is complete and accurate. However, neither the publisher nor the author are engaged in rendering professional advice or services to the individual reader. The ideas, procedures, and suggestions contained in the book are not intended as a substitute for consultation with your healthcare provider. All matters regarding the health of you and your child require medical supervision. Neither the publisher nor the author accept any legal responsibility for any personal injury or other damage or loss arising from the use or misuse of the information and advice in this book.

First published in Great Britain in 2014 by
Dorling Kindersley Limited,
80 Strand, London, WC2R 0RL

A Penguin Random House Company

2 4 6 8 10 9 7 5 3 1
001 – 192071 – Feb/2014
Copyright © 2014 Dorling Kindersley Limited

A CIP catalogue record for this book is available from the British Library.

ISBN 978-1-4093-3751-5

Printed and bound in China by South China Printing Co. Ltd

Discover more at **www.dk.com**

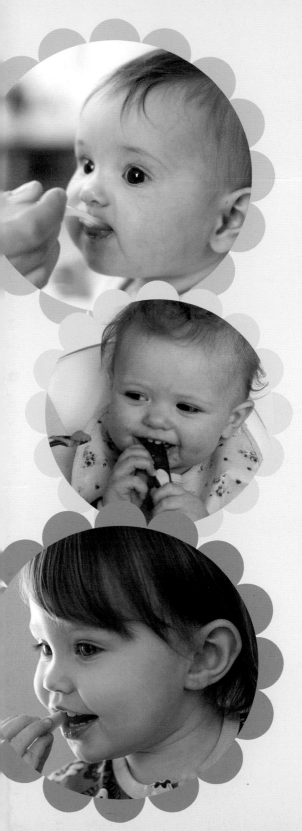

Contents

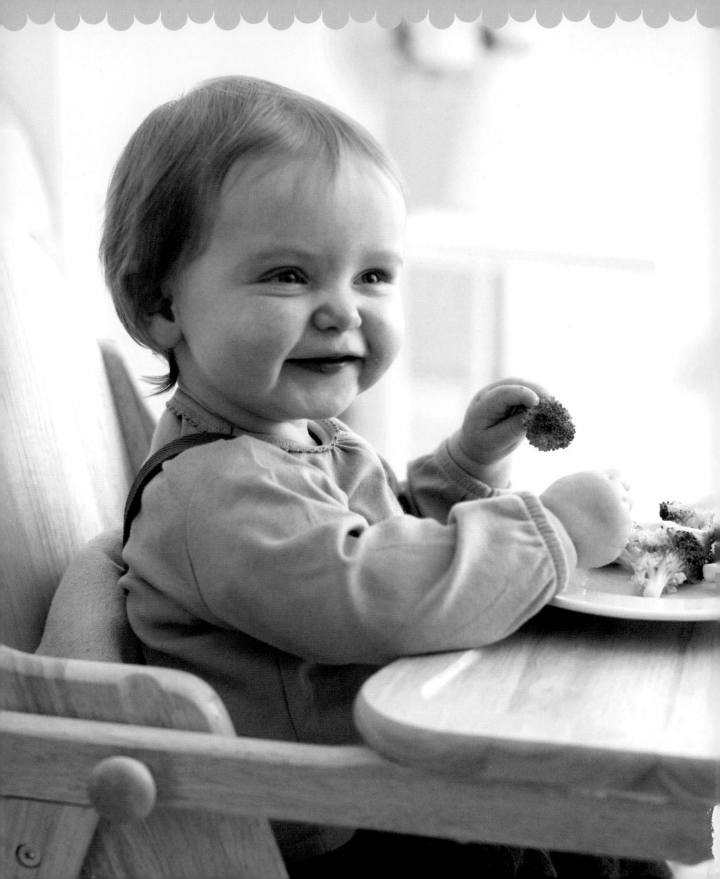

Introduction

It's nearly 20 years since my daughter was born, when the prevailing advice was to wait until four months to introduce any "solid" foods into a baby's diet, and then to opt for baby rice first. In the intervening years, our understanding of both the science and psychology of feeding babies and children has improved, and the guidelines have changed alongside it.

However, in the work I do, and with the parents and babies I meet, I am still aware that whatever the guidelines are, this new stage in a baby's life can be a daunting time for parents, as they try to "get it right". Guidelines are, of course, written for populations, and each individual baby will have his or her own needs.

In writing this book, I have tried to unpack the science and psychology that are behind dietary recommendations by providing simple and practical advice and suggestions for parents. Where there are areas of debate, I've included details so that you can make an informed decision about what you choose to do.

This book contains 200 fully tested recipes for the various stages and styles of weaning, and these provide a progression of flavours and textures. So a parent starting with purées can try a host of delicious simple recipes from first tastes to more complex dishes, and a parent following a baby-led weaning approach will find plenty of nutritious suitable handleable foods for her baby. Whichever method you use, the aim is the same – to have your baby eating a wide range of nutritious foods and joining in with family meals by the time her first birthday arrives.

I've devised menu plans from the first day of weaning right up to and beyond your baby's first birthday. These menu plans provide you with meals, ideas, and alternatives for each meal, making sure that each week your baby is exposed to new flavours and foods. They have been designed so that your baby has a great balance of different vegetables and fruits, learns to eat fish, poultry, and meat, enjoys dairy-based meals and desserts, and tries different types of beans, grains, and potatoes. Foods that have been introduced in a simple form early on are repeated over the weeks, so that your baby has multiple exposure to nutritious foods, which evidence shows is a great way to engender good eating habits for life.

The menu plans have been devised to provide a wide range of nutrients to cover the needs of many babies. I don't claim that 100 per cent of the vitamin E your baby needs on any particular Tuesday will be supplied by that day's meals, as each recipe has not been individually analyzed for its nutrition content. However, I have used my experience as a nutritionist in feeding babies to put together the recipes and menu plans in a way that should provide great nutrition as well as enjoyable eating. Of course, the menu plans don't need to be followed rigidly. They are there if you want clear guidance or they may form the backbone of a weekly eating plan. Or you may prefer to use them for inspiration or ideas alone.

So I wish you fun as you start on this exciting journey, introducing your child to the world of food, and hope that this book will help you on your way.

Fiona Wilcock

About this book

Feeding Your Baby Day by Day starts with essential information on how to go about weaning your baby, then gives practical week-by-week meal planners followed by recipe sections organized by age and stage.

Menu planners

There is a meal planner for each week of weaning in stages 1, 2, and 3. In the last section of the book, there is also a two-week sample planner full of ideas for family meals for the over ones. Every meal in the menu planners can be found in the recipe sections – cross references are given to help you to locate the recipes easily.

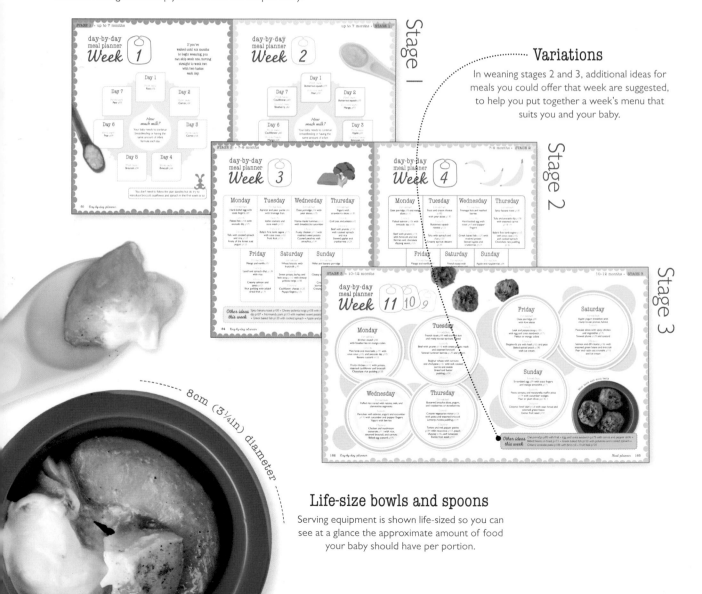

Variations

In weaning stages 2 and 3, additional ideas for meals you could offer that week are suggested, to help you put together a week's menu that suits you and your baby.

Life-size bowls and spoons

Serving equipment is shown life-sized so you can see at a glance the approximate amount of food your baby should have per portion.

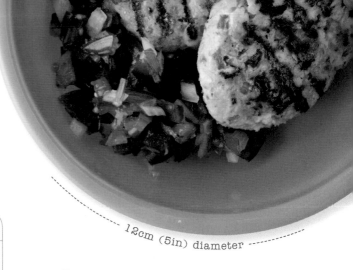

Recipes

The recipe pages are ordered from light meals through to main meals and puddings, so it's easy to navigate your way around the recipes, and reference this section independently of the menu planners if you wish.

There is no need to stop cooking recipes for younger babies once your baby has moved on to the next weaning stage. If your baby has some firm favourites, you can continue to cook these, simply adjusting the texture as necessary to suit your older baby.

Recipe Key

 Preparation time

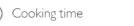 Cooking time

 No cooking required

 Number of portions

Suitable for freezing

...... 12cm (5in) diameter ......

Portion sizes ......

For the more complex recipes, the number of both adult and baby portions is given, making it easier for you to share the meal with your baby.

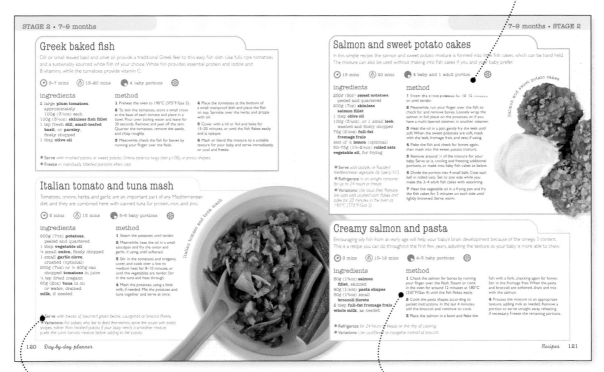

STAGE 2 · 7–9 months

Greek baked fish

Dill or small leaved basil and olive oil provide a traditional Greek feel to this easy fish dish. Use fully ripe tomatoes and a sustainably sourced white fish of your choice. White fish provides essential protein and iodine and B vitamins, while the tomatoes provide vitamin C.

5–7 mins   15–20 mins   4 baby portions

ingredients
2 large **plum tomatoes**, approximately 100g (3½oz) each
100g (3½oz) **skinless fish fillet**
1 tsp fresh **dill**, **small-leafed basil**, or **parsley**, finely chopped
1 tbsp **olive oil**

method
1 Preheat the oven to 190°C (375°F/Gas 5).
2 To skin the tomatoes, score a small cross at the base of each tomato and place in a bowl. Pour over boiling water and leave for 30 seconds. Remove and peel off the skin. Quarter the tomatoes, remove the seeds, and chop roughly.
3 Meanwhile, check the fish for bones by running your finger over the flesh.
4 Place the tomatoes at the bottom of a small ovenproof dish and place the fish on top. Sprinkle over the herbs and drizzle with oil.
5 Cover with a lid or foil and bake for 15–20 minutes, or until the fish flakes easily and is opaque.
6 Mash or blend the mixture to a suitable texture for your baby and serve immediately, or cool and freeze.

✱ Serve with mashed potato or sweet potato. Cheesy polenta twigs (see p.108), or pasta shapes.
✱ Freeze in individually labelled portions when cool.

Italian tomato and tuna mash

Tomatoes, onions, herbs, and garlic are an important part of any Mediterranean diet, and they are combined here with canned tuna for protein, iron, and zinc.

5 mins   15 mins   5–6 baby portions

ingredients
200g (7oz) **potatoes**, peeled and quartered
1 tbsp **vegetable oil**
¼ small **onion**, finely chopped
1 small **garlic clove**, crushed (optional)
200g (7oz) or ½ 400g can chopped **tomatoes** in juice
¼ tsp dried **oregano**
60g (2oz) **tuna** in oil or water, drained
milk, if needed

method
1 Steam the potatoes until tender.
2 Meanwhile, heat the oil in a small saucepan and fry the onion and garlic, if using, until softened.
3 Stir in the tomatoes and oregano, cover, and cook over a low to medium heat for 8–10 minutes, or until the vegetables are tender. Stir in the tuna and heat through.
4 Mash the potatoes, using a little milk, if needed. Mix the potatoes and tuna together and serve at once.

✱ Serve with pieces of steamed green beans, courgettes or broccoli florets.
✱ Variations: For babies who like to feed themselves, serve the sauce with pasta shapes, rather than mashed potato. If your baby needs a smoother mixture, purée the tuna-tomato mixture before adding to the potato.

Italian tomato and tuna mash

7–9 months · STAGE 2

Salmon and sweet potato cakes

In this simple recipe, the salmon and sweet potato mixture is formed into light fish cakes, which can be hand held. The mixture can also be used without making into fish cakes if you and your baby prefer.

15 mins   20 mins   4 baby and 1 adult portion

ingredients
250g (9oz) **sweet potatoes** peeled and quartered
200g (7oz) **skinless salmon fillet**
1 tbsp **olive oil**
100g (3½oz), or 1 small **leek**, washed and finely chopped
75g (2½oz) **full-fat fromage frais**
zest of ½ **lemon** (optional)
50–75g (1¾–2½oz) **rolled oats**
vegetable oil, for frying

method
1 Steam the sweet potatoes for 10–15 minutes, or until tender.
2 Meanwhile, run your finger over the fish to check for and remove bones. Loosely wrap the salmon in foil, place on the potatoes, or, if you have a multi-layered steamer, in another steamer.
3 Heat the oil in a pan, gently fry the leek until soft. When the sweet potatoes are soft, mash with the leek, fromage frais, and zest, if using.
4 Flake the fish and check for bones again, then mash into the sweet potato mixture.
5 Remove around ¼ of the mixture for your baby. Serve as is, cooling and freezing additional portions, or make into baby fish cakes as below.
6 Divide the portion into 4 small balls. Coat each ball in rolled oats. Set to one side while you make the 3–4 adult fish cakes with seasoning.
7 Heat the vegetable oil in a frying pan and fry the fish cakes for 5 minutes on each side until lightly browned. Serve warm.

✱ Serve with tzatziki, or Roasted Mediterranean vegetable dip (see p.107).
✱ Refrigerate in an airtight container for up to 24 hours or freeze.
✱ Variations: Use trout fillet. Reduce the oats with crushed corn flakes and bake for 20 minutes in the oven at 190°C (375°F/Gas 5).

Salmon and sweet potato cakes

Creamy salmon and pasta

Encouraging oily fish from an early age will help your baby's brain development because of the omega 3 content. This is a recipe you can do throughout the first few years, adjusting the texture as your baby is more able to chew.

3 mins   10–12 mins   4–6 baby portions

ingredients
80g (1¾oz) **salmon fillet**, skinned
40g (1½oz) **pasta shapes**
80g (1¾oz) small **broccoli florets**
2 tbsp **full-fat fromage frais**
whole milk, as needed

method
1 Check the salmon for bones by running your finger over the flesh. Steam or cook in the oven for around 12 minutes at 180°C (350°F/Gas 4) until the fish flakes easily.
2 Cook the pasta shapes according to packet instructions. In the last 4 minutes, add the broccoli and continue to cook.
3 Place the salmon in a bowl and flake the fish with a fork, checking again for bones. Stir in the fromage frais. When the pasta and broccoli are softened, drain and mix with the salmon.
4 Process the mixture to an appropriate texture, adding milk as needed. Remove a portion to serve straight away, reheating if necessary. Freeze the remaining portions.

✱ Refrigerate for 24 hours or freeze on the day of cooking.
✱ Variations: Use cauliflower or courgette instead of broccoli.

Serving, storage, and variations

Serving suggestions are provided at the end of recipes, as is guidance on cooling and how long food can be refrigerated or frozen for. Recipe variations are also given sometimes, helping you to take account of seasonal availability and tastes.

...... Oven temperatures

Temperatures are given in celsius, with fahrenheit and gas conversions. If you have a fan-assisted oven, reduce the celsius temperature by 20°C; for example, a recipe that requires an oven temperature of 190°C would be 170°C for a fan-assisted oven.

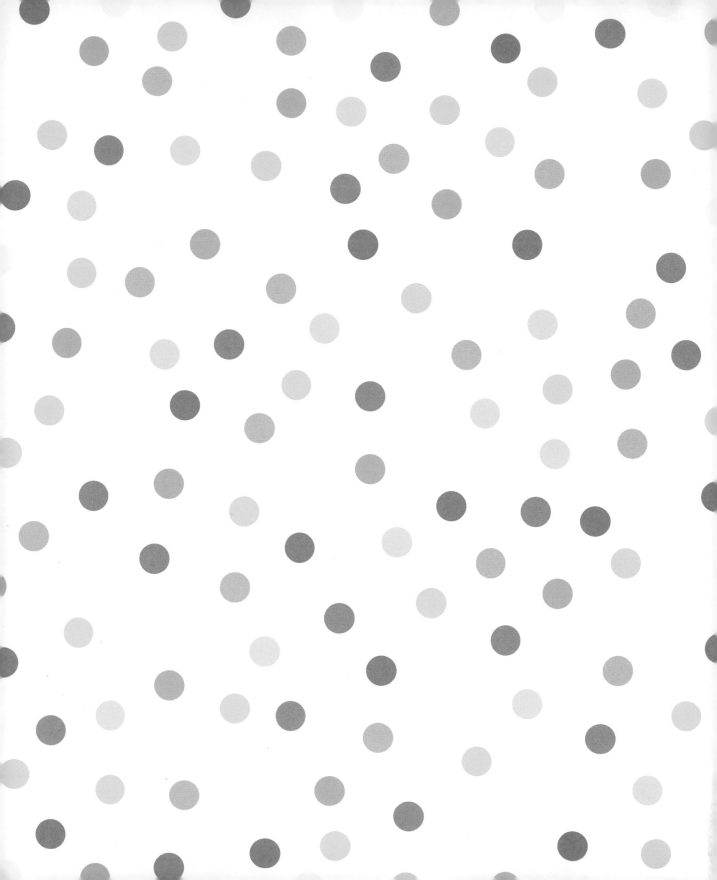

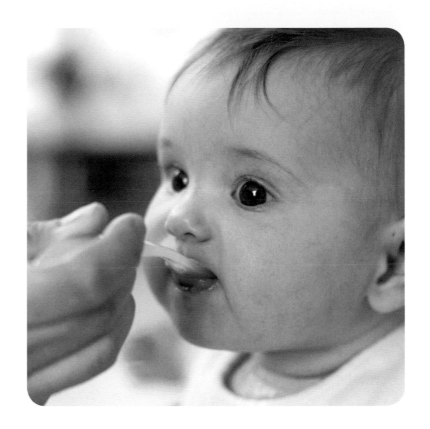

Welcome to *weaning!*

Weaning your baby means starting to give her solid foods alongside her usual milk feeds. By the time your baby is a year old, she should be able to take part in your family meals. To find out everything you need to know, including when to start and what to do, read on.

Is your baby *ready?*

All babies grow and develop at different rates. However, whether your baby was born early or late, struggled to establish breastfeeding, or sailed through the early weeks, there are some important developmental signs to look out for, usually present between four and six months, that indicate she is probably ready to start being weaned onto solid foods.

Perfect timing

Working out the best time to wean your baby can make a difference to how smoothly the process goes. Most babies are weaned between 17 weeks and six months; every baby is an individual and there is no one-size-fits-all rule as to when exactly to start your baby on solids. You do need to make sure your baby is showing the developmental signs shown opposite. Be guided by your baby and talk to your GP or health visitor if you're unsure whether she is ready, especially if she was premature (see pp34–5).

Never start weaning before 17 weeks of age. Before this age, your baby isn't able to process foods properly because her kidneys and digestive system are too immature. It's also inadvisable to leave it later than six months as by then your baby needs more nutrients than milk alone provides.

If you are breastfeeding, continuing to do so while weaning is thought to be beneficial, especially if you start weaning before six months. There is some evidence that babies who are breastfed alongside first solids (including allergenic foods such as wheat) before six months of age (but not before 17 weeks), are less likely to develop coeliac disease, type 1 diabetes, or wheat allergy.

One of the main goals of the weaning process is to teach your baby to fit in with your healthy family meals.

What's the official line?

You may find yourself confused by contradictory official guidelines, as many governments advise exclusive breastfeeding for the first six months of life. This advice stems from the World Health Organization (WHO) and is based on the beneficial effects of breastfeeding in countries where poor hygiene makes this the safest option, as well as on the positive long-term effects of breast milk. Some experts, though, think the WHO guidelines are not as relevant in developed countries. They highlight that breast milk alone doesn't supply enough iron and zinc for a baby by the time she is six months old, especially if she was 2.5kg (5lb 8oz) or more at birth.

A window of opportunity

When you decide to start weaning may be influenced by the so-called "window of opportunity". Child psychologists suggest that babies who are developmentally ready and start weaning between four and six months accept new tastes and textures more readily than those weaned later. This period, which extends to seven months, is seen as a chance to expand your baby's diet. If you wean at six months, you need to introduce new flavours more quickly, and move more rapidly on to lumps and finger foods.

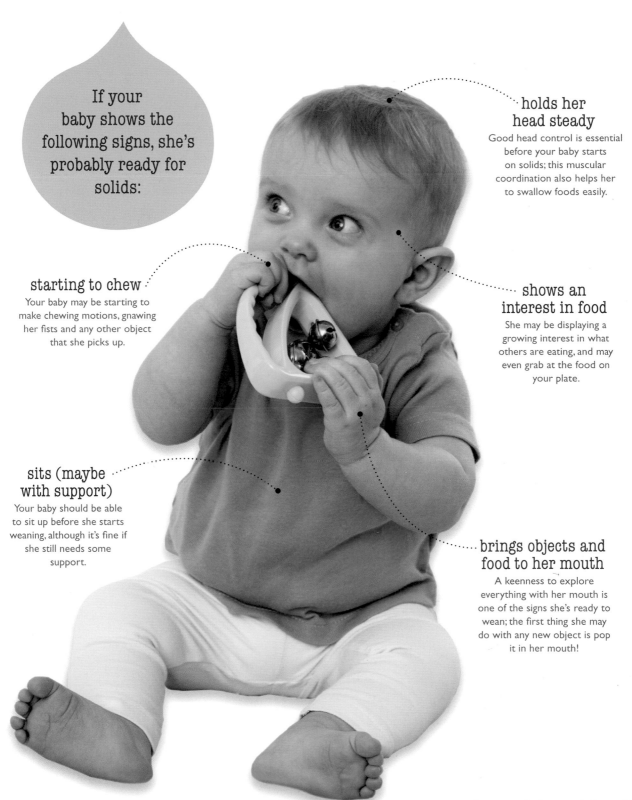

If your baby shows the following signs, she's probably ready for solids:

holds her head steady
Good head control is essential before your baby starts on solids; this muscular coordination also helps her to swallow foods easily.

starting to chew
Your baby may be starting to make chewing motions, gnawing her fists and any other object that she picks up.

shows an interest in food
She may be displaying a growing interest in what others are eating, and may even grab at the food on your plate.

sits (maybe with support)
Your baby should be able to sit up before she starts weaning, although it's fine if she still needs some support.

brings objects and food to her mouth
A keenness to explore everything with her mouth is one of the signs she's ready to wean; the first thing she may do with any new object is pop it in her mouth!

Your baby's *changing* diet

Milk dominates your baby's diet throughout the first year, whether you are breast- or formula feeding, but by six months of age, her needs for growth and development are no longer met by milk alone.

Complementary, or weaning, foods are introduced to provide essential nutrients and different tastes and textures. Accepting new textures enhances your baby's learning of key skills such as chewing and speech development. As more foods are introduced and the quantity increases, some milk is naturally displaced, so what constitutes a balanced diet at five months will be different from one at eight or 12 months, as solids become more important. As your

baby approaches one year, the amount of milk she drinks each day will have decreased from around a litre (1¾ pints) of formula, or breastfeeding on demand, to 400–500ml (13½–17fl oz) formula, or two to three breastfeeds a day.

Once your baby has got used to first tastes, she needs to eat foods from the same four main food groups as you, however, the quantities and proportions are different to meet her high requirements for energy and nutrients.

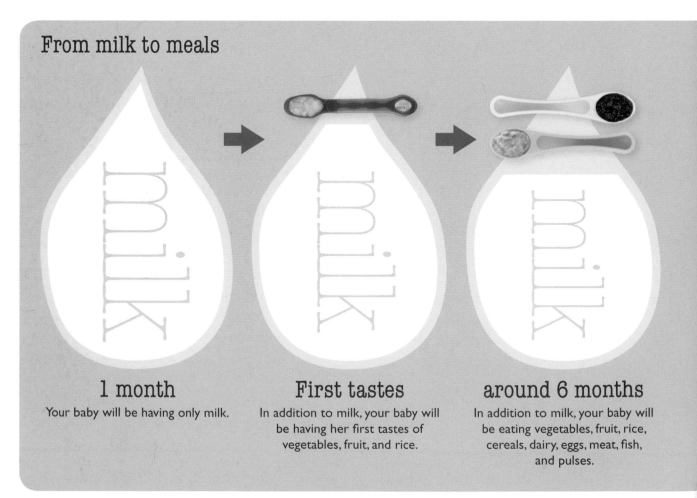

From milk to meals

1 month
Your baby will be having only milk.

First tastes
In addition to milk, your baby will be having her first tastes of vegetables, fruit, and rice.

around 6 months
In addition to milk, your baby will be eating vegetables, fruit, rice, cereals, dairy, eggs, meat, fish, and pulses.

Milk and dairy foods

Full-fat milk, full-fat, unsweetened yogurt and fromage frais, and hard cheeses provide calories and protein as well as essential vitamins and minerals such as calcium, zinc, and magnesium.

Bread, cereals, and potatoes

These starchy foods provide calories, B vitamins, and some iron. While wholegrain is good for adults, too much fibre can fill up your baby's tummy, not leaving enough space for other more nutritious foods. White bread, pasta, and rice are fine for babies; offer wholegrain occasionally, gradually introducing more during the toddler and preschool years.

 ## Meat, poultry, fish, eggs, and pulses

These foods provide protein, minerals, especially iron and zinc, fatty acids (from fish), and B vitamins.

Vegetables and fruit

These provide vitamins, minerals, dietary fibre, and plant chemicals, sometimes called phytochemicals, such as antioxidants that protect the body from disease.

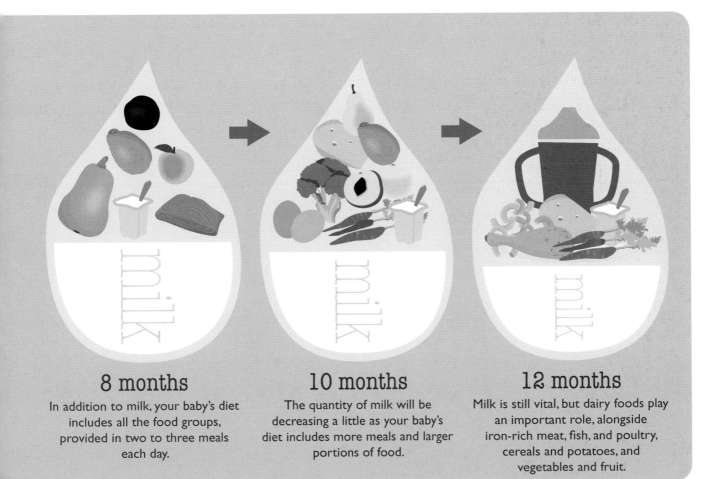

8 months
In addition to milk, your baby's diet includes all the food groups, provided in two to three meals each day.

10 months
The quantity of milk will be decreasing a little as your baby's diet includes more meals and larger portions of food.

12 months
Milk is still vital, but dairy foods play an important role, alongside iron-rich meat, fish, and poultry, cereals and potatoes, and vegetables and fruit.

Food for *growing*

Each food contains a mixture of different nutrients, which have a range of functions to help your baby grow and develop. Some of the main nutrients that contribute to different areas of development are shown below. Some foods are especially good sources of particular nutrients, as shown on pages 16–17.

For healthy growth:

Protein is the building block for every cell in your baby's body, and protein-rich foods are essential for her to grow and develop normally.

Iron forms part of the red blood cells that transport oxygen around the body. Too little iron causes anaemia, which may cause delays in development and growth. By six months, your breast milk and the iron reserves your baby was born with no longer provide adequate iron, so providing iron-rich foods is important. In toddlers, anaemia can be traced back to a poor weaning diet.

Vitamin B2 helps to keep the skin healthy.

Vitamin C helps in the formation of your child's blood vessels, muscles, cartilage, and bone.

Vitamin E is essential for the formation of red blood cells, muscles, and tissues, and also helps to keep the skin healthy.

For the eyes, brain, and nervous system:

Omega 3 fatty acids are essential polyunsaturated fatty acids for the development of your baby's brain, vision, and nervous system.

Vitamin A helps the healthy development of your baby's eyes.

Vitamin B12 helps the development and working of your baby's nervous system.

Folic acid is essential for the nervous system and brain.

For energy:

Carbohydrates are sugars and starch that supply essential energy for your baby. Your baby doesn't need added sugars in her diet; sugars occur naturally in many foods including milk (breast milk is naturally sweet), fruits, and vegetables.

Fats are a concentrated source of energy (calories), which is perfect for your baby as she can eat only small amounts of food at a time. Around half of the calories in breast or formula milk come from fat, so it's important not to drop milk feeds when you start solids because your baby needs these for energy. As more foods are introduced, include small quantities of high-fat foods. Low- or reduced-fat foods aren't suitable for babies.

B vitamins help your baby release energy from carbohydrates and fats.

For strong bones and teeth:

Calcium is essential for the healthy growth and development of your baby's bones and teeth. For the first few months, breast and formula milk supply this mineral, and although milk continues to be an important source, other calcium-rich foods need to be added to your baby's daily diet as you begin weaning, especially as the amount of milk gradually decreases.

Vitamin D has a wide range of protective roles and also works alongside calcium to help in the formation of your baby's teeth and bones. Babies who have inadequate vitamin D in the first year of life can develop the bone-softening disease rickets. As their bones aren't properly formed, this affects them when they start to stand or walk. Most vitamin D comes from the action of sunlight on the skin, and the body stores some for less sunny months. Rickets has started to recur in parts of the developed world as children spend less time outdoors exposed to sunshine. Very few foods contain much vitamin D, although some foods including infant breakfast cereals are now fortified with it.

Vitamin A helps strong growth in your baby's bones.

For a healthy immune system and good healing:

Zinc is a mineral that helps promote growth, boosts the immune system, and helps wounds to heal. In the UK, many toddlers do not have sufficient zinc, which can cause growth problems, so including foods with zinc in your baby's diet in the first year is important.

Vitamin C plays an important role in preventing infection as well as healing.

Vitamin A helps resist and fight infection. Some babies and toddlers don't have enough vitamin A, which makes them more prone to infections and other complications.

Vitamin E is an important, widely found, vitamin that promotes healing.

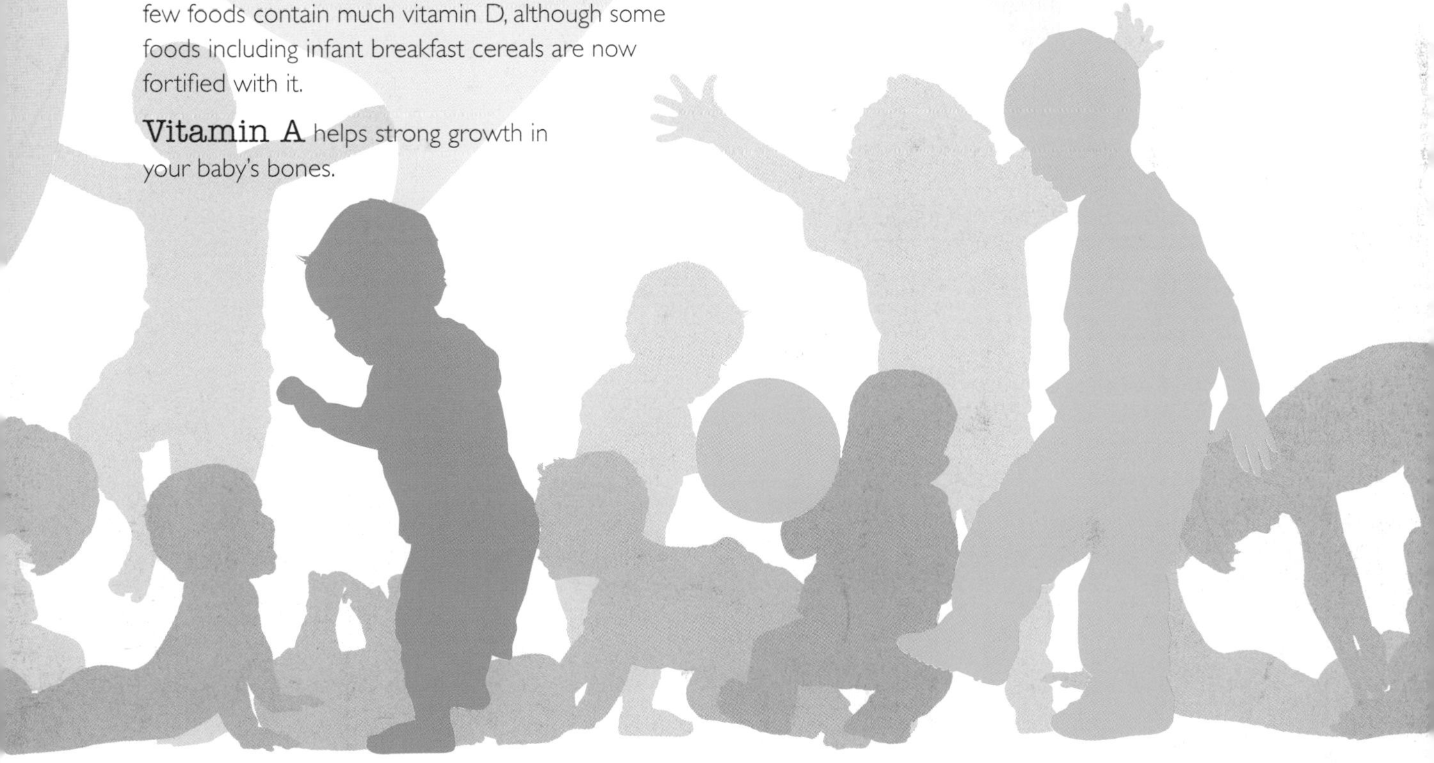

Know your *nutrients!*

Each food your baby eats is made up of various nutrients, including essential vitamins and minerals, so providing a range of healthy foods will help your baby flourish. The boxes below list the best sources of nutrients first. The meal planners in the book are designed to provide a healthy, balanced diet for your baby.

Fats

SOURCES

- Oily fish, such as salmon, mackerel, and sardines
- Full-fat dairy: cheese, yogurt, and milk *
- Meat
- Oils, such as rapeseed, olive, and vegetable
- Seeds and nuts (not whole)

Fats are composed of a mixture of different types of fatty acids. Vegetable oils, seeds, and nuts contain more monounsaturated and polyunsaturated fatty acids, which are better for us than saturated fats, more commonly found in processed foods, dairy, and fatty meats. "Trans" fats, which are more likely to be found in lower-quality processed food, are particularly unhealthy.

Omega 3 fatty acids

SOURCES

- Oily fish, such as salmon, mackerel, and sardines
- Fish oil supplements [+]
- Nuts and seeds
- Vegetable oils

The particularly good omega 3s are naturally present in fish oils. The other types of omega 3s from plant sources have to be converted in the body to the more useful type.

Carbohydrates
(includes starches and sugars)

SOURCES

- Bread
- Potatoes
- Rice and other grains
- Cereals
- Fruits
- Vegetables
- Milk *
- Yogurt

Proteins

SOURCES

- Milk *
- Eggs
- Meat
- Poultry
- Fish
- Pulses
- Tofu, quorn, or soya
- Nut and seed butters

Iron

SOURCES

- Canned sardines and pilchards
- Liver **
- Lean beef, lamb, and pork
- Dark cuts of chicken or turkey such as thigh
- Sausages
- Fish paste
- Fortified breakfast cereals
- Eggs
- Bread
- Beans, especially red kidney and haricot
- Baked beans
- Tofu
- Dried fruit: prunes, figs, raisins, and sultanas
- Cauliflower, broccoli, and spring greens

There are two types of iron, one found in animal foods, the other in plant foods. Iron from animal sources is more easily absorbed. Vitamin C helps the absorption of iron from plant sources, so if your baby has little or no meat, try giving a cup of unsweetened fruit juice, diluted one part juice to 10 parts water at mealtimes.

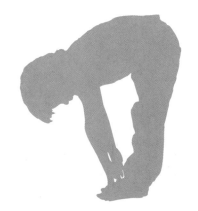

Calcium

SOURCES

- Hard cheeses and soya "cheese"
- Canned fish with bones mashed (sardines or salmon)
- Tofu
- Milk *
- Yogurt
- White bread or products from white flour
- Dairy ice cream
- Beans, lentils, and chickpeas
- Squash and sweet potato
- Broccoli, spinach, and kale
- Peas
- Dates, sultanas, and ready-to-eat apricots

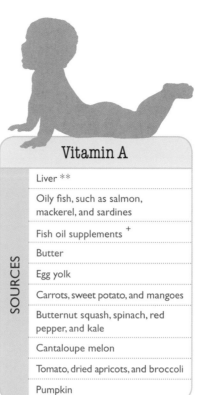

Vitamin A

SOURCES

- Liver **
- Oily fish, such as salmon, mackerel, and sardines
- Fish oil supplements +
- Butter
- Egg yolk
- Carrots, sweet potato, and mangoes
- Butternut squash, spinach, red pepper, and kale
- Cantaloupe melon
- Tomato, dried apricots, and broccoli
- Pumpkin

Vitamin C

SOURCES

- Red pepper and blackcurrants
- Strawberries
- Brussel sprouts and kiwi fruit
- Oranges, clementines, and mangoes
- Nectarines and raspberries
- Grapefruit
- Papaya
- Cauliflower
- Swede
- Cabbage
- New potatoes
- Pineapple and peas

Vitamin D

SOURCES

- Oily fish, such as salmon, mackerel, and sardines
- Eggs
- Fortified breakfast cereals
- Butter and spreads

Vitamin B2

SOURCES

- Liver **
- Fortified breakfast cereals
- Cheese
- Almonds (ground)
- Milk *

Vitamin E

SOURCES

- Vegetable oils
- Nuts and seeds
- Avocado
- Eggs

Zinc

SOURCES

- Quorn
- Fish
- Meat
- Nut and seed butters
- Wholegrains
- Eggs
- Milk *

Vitamin B12

SOURCES

- Liver **
- Fish
- Meat
- Eggs

Folic acid

SOURCES

- Liver **
- Fortified breakfast cereals
- Broccoli
- Brussels sprouts and spinach
- Pinto and black-eyed beans
- Beetroot and oranges

---

* Don't use cow's milk as a drink before 12 months.

** Liver is so high in vitamin A, it is normally not recommended under one year. If given, this should be occasionally only.

\+ Only use fish oil supplements that are suitable for babies and children, and not if you are using formula. Seek advice from your doctor.

Best for baby

Encouraging your baby to eat well from an early age helps her to grow and develop into a healthy toddler and child, and has a positive long-term impact on her health and wellbeing. As well as making sure that your baby's diet includes different food groups that contain essential vitamins and minerals, getting her diet right is also about being aware of some other, often very particular, dietary requirements that apply to young babies.

Avoid adding sugar unnecessarily

Why?

Excess sugar in the diet can lead to tooth decay, and encourage your baby to develop a liking for sweet food over savoury early on, which long-term could lead to obesity and nutrient deficiencies.

What to watch out for: If you breastfeed, up until weaning, your baby has been used to the sweet taste of your milk. As you start to introduce solids, it's important that she learns to accept savoury tastes, so foods shouldn't be sweetened with sugar. Research also suggests that it's best if you don't mix sweet and savoury foods either, so your baby learns to enjoy individual flavours.

Make sure that foods you buy don't contain added sugar. This can come in various guises including honey (which should be avoided before 12 months); sucrose, glucose or fructose syrups; golden syrup; brown, cane or beet sugar; and fruit juice concentrates, to name a few.

White bread, pasta, and rice are fine for babies

Use wholegrain foods occasionally, and gradually introduce more during the toddler and preschool years.

Why?

Foods that are full of fibre (which helps digestion and promotes good health), such as vegetables, fruits, and wholegrains, tend to be quite bulky and don't provide much energy for your baby. This is great if you are a mum watching her weight, but bad news for a baby because her little tummy becomes full of low-calorie fibre, which doesn't provide enough energy or other nutrients for her to grow, and leaves less room for other more nutritious foods.

What to watch out for: Fruits and vegetables provide many essential nutrients, so it's a question of getting the balance right. Too many high-fibre foods can displace other nutritious foods such as dairy foods, meat, fish, eggs, and healthy oils. If as a family you eat only wholemeal bread, this is okay for your baby as long as she isn't having a lot of other fibre-rich foods such as lentils and pulses.

Never add salt to your baby's food

Be aware, too, of hidden salts in other ingredients such as cured meats, smoked fish, brine-preserved ingredients, and high-salt cheeses.

Why?

Salt can overload your baby's developing kidneys, so it's important not to add any to her food. Salt is naturally present in many foods and your baby's requirements are more than met by these. Although her food may not taste as you would like it, it is perfect for her needs.

What to watch out for: Be cautious about using ingredients that are high in salt for family meals you are intending your older baby to share. If necessary, add ingredients such as bacon and cured meats, smoked fish, or olives and other brine-preserved foods to the main dish after her portion has been served and is cooling.

Look at ingredients on food labels and choose those lowest in salt. Use fish or vegetables canned in water or oil, not brine; avoid high-salt cheeses such as Parmesan; and buy salt-free tomato purées and pastes.

Savoury snacks, such as crisps and potato or corn shapes, are very salty and are unsuitable for babies.

Not for babies

There are a few other foods that should be avoided in your baby's first year:

- Honey, due to the small risk of a food poisoning bacterium that can cause infant botulism
- Whole nuts because of the risk of choking
- Shellfish, due to the risk of food poisoning
- Shark, marlin, and swordfish, which may contain mercury or other potential toxins
- Liver, due to its very high vitamin A content
- Unpasteurized cheeses or dairy products
- Diet, or reduced-fat or -sugar, foods or drink.

Organic or non-organic?

Organic farms use fewer chemicals, but is organic food nutritionally better? Evidence is varied and depends on the type of food, the season, even how long a farm has been organic, but it's thought that mostly it doesn't provide more nutrients.

If you buy fresh organic food, bear in mind the shelf life is shorter and wash it carefully before use.

Products grown for commercial baby food are stringently regulated, and therefore there's little, if any, difference between organic and non-organic products.

Do babies need vitamin supplements?

Supplements of vitamins A, D, and C are important for babies with a limited diet, fussy eaters, and for those who don't drink 500ml (17fl oz) of formula milk a day. If you are breastfeeding, you're advised to take a 10mcg vitamin D supplement. Also, Asian, Middle Eastern, and African babies in the UK need vitamin D supplements because they may not make sufficient vitamin D from sunlight.

What's your *style?*

The most usual method of weaning is to start with puréed foods, gradually adapting textures and adding tastes. Another approach, known as baby-led weaning, concentrates on babies feeding themselves whole foods from the outset, starting at six months. Whichever method you follow, the aim is the same: for your baby to be eating healthy, balanced meals with the rest of the family by 12 months of age.

Weaning with purées

For many cultures, weaning starts with giving a baby puréed food from a spoon. The texture of the food varies, starting with runny purées, progressing through to mashed food, food with soft lumps, soft finger foods, and then minced and chopped foods with harder finger foods. At each stage, your baby learns something new and develops new skills. The aim is that by one year she will be able to eat chopped versions of suitable family meals, have started to self-feed using a spoon and/or fingers, and be drinking from a cup (with or without a spout). She will have had the opportunity to try repeatedly a wide range of different foods from all the main food groups, and been part of family meals and social eating occasions.

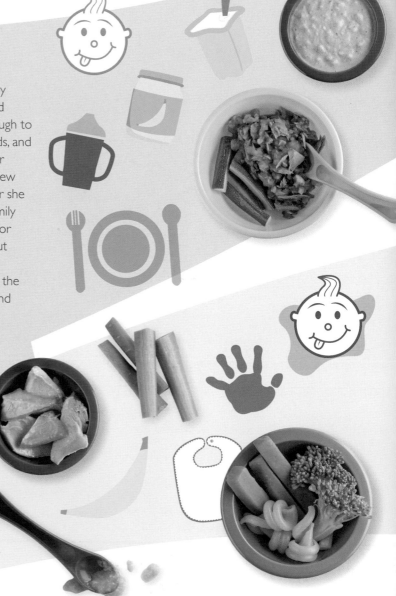

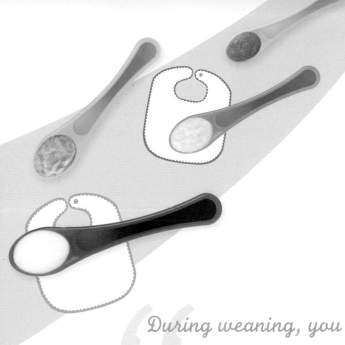

> *During weaning, you introduce your baby gradually to the foods she will eat throughout her life.*

Baby-led weaning (BLW)

This method promotes offering whole cooked foods or soft raw foods rather than puréed foods to your baby, and allows her to feed herself from the outset rather than being spoon-fed by you. BLW allows your baby to take the lead in deciding which foods to try when. It is often said to be a more relaxed, if messy, approach to weaning as babies can enjoy feeling, squishing, and playing with the food as well as eating it.

Advocates claim that it results in children being less fussy about food and better able to control their appetite, which may reduce their risk of becoming overweight, although this has yet to be confirmed by research.

How do you choose?

There are pros and cons to both weaning methods. The more usual purée route is tried and tested, and research shows that it works nutritionally and developmentally. The danger is that babies may struggle moving from purées to lumps if kept on runny purées for too long.

Babies following the BLW route need sufficient hand–eye coordination to pick up food, which ties in with current recommendations to delay weaning to six months. However, there is less research on BLW, and claims that this approach reduces fussy eating later on are yet to be established. It is also not known if babies get adequate nutrition at first, especially of iron, so if you adopt this approach, you still need to ensure that your baby's diet is nutritious and balanced, rather than simply giving foods you happen to be eating.

Your decision may be influenced by your personalities and your baby's abilities. You and your baby may be temperamentally more suited to controlled purée feeding: she may prefer to be spoon-fed until she gains more confidence, and you may appreciate the structure. Alternatively, if your baby has good hand–eye coordination and is independent, she may want to hold a spoon or a piece of food, so if you're happy with the extra mess of BLW, this may work well. There is no reason why you can't combine weaning approaches, or you may wish to try one or the other method first, then work out what suits you both best.

As *easy as* 1, 2, 3...

Weaning is usually described in three stages. During each stage, as well as trying out new foods and textures, your baby develops new skills that help her to eat solids. She learns how to use her tongue, to swallow different textured purées, to chew up and down then in a rotary fashion, and to pick up food and move it to her mouth. She also learns to use her lips to move food from a spoon and to drink from a cup.

Stage 1 — up to 7 months

In the first stage, your baby learns:

- to take food from a spoon by closing her mouth around it
- to move food from the front to the back of her mouth to swallow
- that foods taste different
- to accept purées and then mashed foods, and she may try some first finger foods

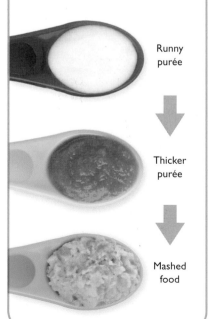

Runny purée

Thicker purée

Mashed food

Stage 2 — from 7 to 9 months

In this stage, your baby learns:

- to move lumps around in her mouth
- to become confident chewing soft lumps
- to use a pincer grip to self-feed soft or dissolving finger foods
- to sip from a cup or beaker with a spout
- to accept a wider range of different foods
- to eat more than one meal a day

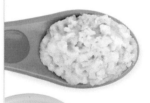

Mashed food

Mashed food with soft lumps

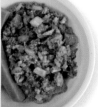

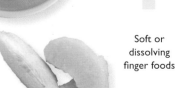

Soft or dissolving finger foods

Stage 3 — from 9 to 12 months

In this stage, your baby learns to:

- master chewing minced and chopped foods
- eat a greater number of finger foods, including those with harder textures
- use her lips to get food off a spoon and become more proficient at self-feeding with a spoon
- curl her lips around a cup or beaker
- accept a wider range of suitable family foods
- eat three meals a day

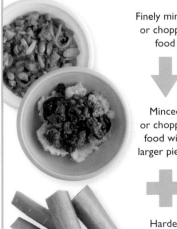

Finely minced or chopped food

Minced or chopped food with larger pieces

Harder finger foods

Baby-led weaning

- If you follow baby-led weaning, starting around six months, your baby will sit with you at mealtimes (whenever possible), and be offered a selection of whole cooked foods or soft fruit, cut into easy-to-handle pieces. She may simply play with the food at first, perhaps suck it, then gradually will start to chew and swallow food.

- If you wish to combine BLW with purée-based weaning, offer soft finger foods alongside purées at around six months.

- You can be led by the planner to ensure your baby receives a balanced diet, cooking and offering the meals chopped rather than puréed or mashed.

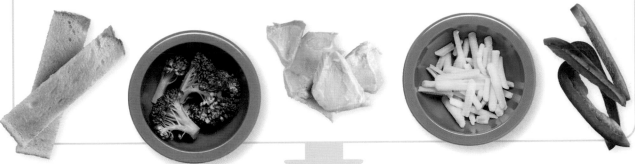

Family meals

By 12 months your baby will:

- be eating chopped up versions of family meals
- eating together with the family whenever possible
- drinking from a lidded cup or beaker

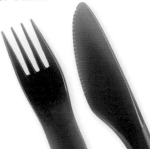

Chopped up family meals

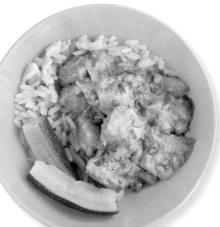

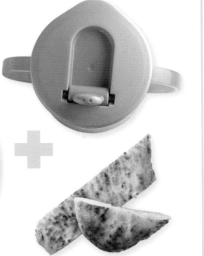

Time to *shop*

Once your baby starts on solids, you will want to be sure that your shopping basket contains storecupboard basics that are suitable for her to eat. Thankfully, many family ingredients are fine for your baby, with just a few that aren't suitable. Knowing which items are okay and which aren't will help you shop with confidence and make the best choices for your baby.

Spreads: full-fat made from olive or sunflower oil.

Cheese: full-fat hard cheese for cooking and full-fat soft cream cheese for spreads and dips.

Oils: monounsaturated vegetable oils, such as rapeseed or olive oil.

Yogurts and fromage frais: plain, full-fat, unsweetened varieties. Sweeten them naturally with home-made purées or stewed fruits.

Cereals: low-sugar and low-salt varieties; iron-fortified.

Frozen vegetables: frozen vegetables, such as chopped spinach, peas, and butternut squash sometimes have a higher nutritional value than fresh versions as they are frozen at their peak condition.

Milk: full-fat cow's milk can be used for cooking after six months. It isn't suitable as a drink before one year as it doesn't provide sufficient iron.

Canned chopped tomatoes or tomato passata: useful when making family meals to share with older babies. Choose varieties with no added sugar or salt.

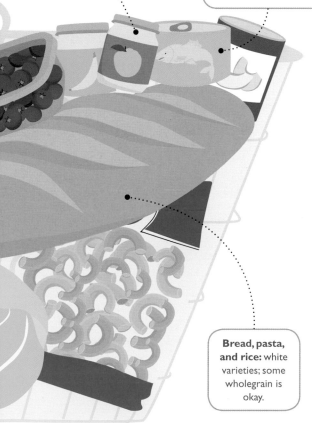

Spices, herbs, ginger, and garlic.

Commercial baby foods: there is a good range of commercial baby foods, with many providing a wide variety of ingredients and nutrients.

Canned foods: opt for fruits preserved in their juices; vegetables, pulses, and beans in water; tuna in water or oil. Cans are convenient and offer a variety of colours and flavours when fresh fruit or vegetables aren't in season.

Bread, pasta, and rice: white varieties; some wholegrain is okay.

Fruits and vegetables: seasonal, in a variety of colours.

Leave it on the shelf!

The following items shouldn't be included in your baby's storecupboard or diet.

- **Fruit juices** provide vitamin C, but they're high in sugars, which can lead to tooth decay and a preference for sweet food. Strictly limit or avoid these, unless your baby is a vegetarian, in which case giving unsweetened fruit juice diluted one part to 10 with water at mealtimes helps iron absorption.

- **Squashes and cordials** also encourage a sweet tooth and can cause tooth decay. Fizzy drinks and artificially sweetened diet drinks intended for adults should definitely be avoided.

- **Drinks containing caffeine** aren't suitable for babies or small children. Tea and coffee are stimulants and contain tannins, which affect the absorption of iron.

- Avoid **salty foods and sauces,** such as soy sauce; tomato ketchup; spicy curry sauces; sauces with added cheese, ham or bacon; chutneys and pickles; cured meats (bacon, salami); crisps, or other savoury snacks; olives preserved in brine; adult ready-meals, and stock cubes.

- **Chilli** isn't suitable for babies.

- Your baby doesn't need **confectionery or sugar**, unless used to sweeten a sour fruit when cooking, so avoid sweet processed foods such as jams, some breakfast cereals, cakes, biscuits, ice creams, and lollies. Custard is okay occasionally, but check that the colour comes only from betacarotene and, if using powdered custard, make it with a minimum of sugar.

- **Goat's or sheep's milk** can be allergenic, and these don't provide sufficient nutrients for your baby under one year.

- **Butter** is high in saturated fat so should be used only sparingly.

Into the *kitchen*

With the right equipment and preparation, making home-made purées is simple. You need to be scrupulous about kitchen hygiene and store food correctly to ensure it stays as fresh as possible. Build in preparation time for chopping and slicing fresh produce and think about quantities too: cooking more than your baby needs for one meal means you can freeze purées and have ready-made meals to hand for busy days.

Safety first

Young babies are more vulnerable to infections than adults so it's vital that you follow good hygiene practice while preparing your baby's food to minimize the risk of transferring germs and infections to your baby.

- Wash your hands with soap before handling food.

- Before and after preparing and cooking your baby's food, wipe surfaces thoroughly with a clean cloth soaked in hot, soapy water to eliminate germs and bacteria. Use disposable cloths or rotate clean cloths daily.

- If you have pets, don't allow them on work surfaces or near foods. Use separate utensils and bowls for pets.

- Wash fruit, vegetables, and potatoes before preparing.

- Cook eggs until solid and meat and poultry until there's no pink flesh and the juices run clear.

Preparing food

Making healthy home-made food for your baby involves quite a bit of preparation time as you peel, chop, and slice fresh produce. You may already have everything you need to do this, but it's worth checking that your knives are sharpened and chopping boards aren't too worn. If you wish, you might want to invest in equipment such as a food processor to help speed up the preparation; there is a range of models available depending on your needs.

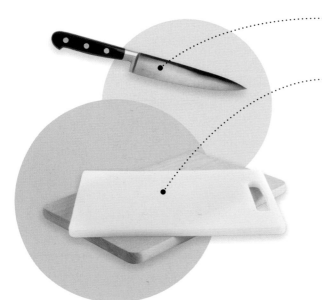

A sharp knife
A properly sharpened knife is a basic essential for efficient home cooking.

Chopping boards
Use separate chopping boards for preparing raw items such as meat and fish, and cooked items or fruit and vegetables to prevent cross-contamination.

Mini chopper
Mini food processors chop small amounts of food quickly. Look for one with more than one speed that enables you to control texture.

Food processor
These can have a variety of functions, including chopping and puréeing, and the cost varies accordingly. If you enjoy cooking, you might want to invest in a more expensive model with discs for grating and slicing.

Batch cooking and freezing

Your baby eats only small quantities of food at a time, so batch cooking and freezing larger quantities avoids wastage and reduces the amount of time you spend in the kitchen. Vitamins are lost during preparation and storage, so chill and freeze foods quickly to minimize losses.

Freezing: Pour hot purées straight into ice-cube trays or small pots, cover, leave to cool thoroughly (not in the fridge), then freeze straightaway. On a hot day, you can place food in sealed pots and pop these into a bowl of cold water with ice cubes to speed up chilling. Label the pot or tray with the content and date and freeze at -18°C/0°F.

Defrosting: The safest way to defrost foods is overnight in the fridge. They can also be defrosted in a bowl in a microwave following the oven instructions. Don't leave foods to defrost at room temperature, particularly if they contain meat or fish.

Reheating: Defrosted food can be reheated in the microwave (or a pan) until it is piping hot, then removed and stirred well to get rid of "hot spots". Cool the food before serving to your baby, checking the temperature by testing a blob on the inside of your wrist: it should feel neither hot nor cold. Cool it for a few more minutes if it's still hot. Reheat defrosted foods once only.

Useful storage items

Lidded plastic pots and ice-cube trays
Lidded plastic pots are handy for storing items in the fridge, keeping them separate from other foods. Individual ice-cube trays or lidded portion pots are ideal for freezing purées as you can defrost just the quantity of ice-cube portions required for one meal.

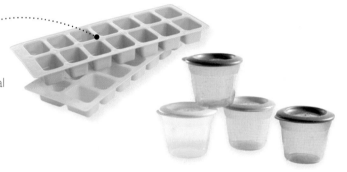

Storing foods

For the fridge, follow these guidelines to keep fresh, perishable produce at its best:

- Set your fridge at 4°C (39.2°F). Use a thermometer if you wish.
- Keep the most perishable foods such as meat, fish, and poultry in the coldest part of the fridge.
- Raw foods such as meat, fish, and poultry should be well wrapped, or put in an airtight container, so they don't drip on other foods.
- Loosely wrap vegetables and fruits in polythene bags.
- Check "use by" dates on foods that go off quickly, such as dairy, fish, and meat; these are unsafe to eat after this date. If a label states an item can be eaten within three days of opening but this passes the use by date, it isn't safe to eat.
- Don't keep food that your baby has half eaten.

In the storecupboard, for non-perishable foods:

- Ensure the cupboard is cool and dry.
- Rotate foods so the first in are eaten first, and follow the instructions for storage on the label.
- Check "best before" dates on foods such as pasta, cereals, and rice. These foods aren't unsafe to eat after this date, but the taste or quality may decline. The exception is eggs, which should be eaten within a couple of days after the "best before" date.

How to make *baby purées*

Cooking baby purées is quite straightforward, and you will probably find that you derive a great deal of pleasure from cooking nutritious food for your baby. Being well-organized, for example ensuring that food is ready before your baby becomes too hungry and upset, will make mealtimes more relaxed. Make sure your ingredients are in peak condition and cook foods thoroughly to avoid food poisoning.

1 Cook the ingredients until just tender

Apart from a few fruits that can be given to your baby raw, most first foods need to be cooked to reduce the risk of food poisoning. Cooking destroys around half of the vitamin C content of food and some B vitamins (more if the water they are cooked in is thrown away), so when possible use methods such as steaming, which preserves the most vitamins and minerals. Sometimes, though, the nutrient content of a food actually improves with cooking. For example, the naturally occurring chemical lycopene, found in tomatoes, which has specific health benefits, is released more readily with cooking. Cooking also makes dietary fibre more digestible.

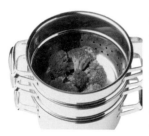

Steaming
This is a good way to cook vegetables and potatoes as it's quicker than boiling and the food doesn't come into contact with water so fewer vitamins and minerals are lost.

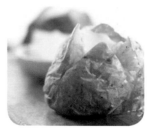

Oven baking
Some fruits or vegetables can be softened by oven baking, which is an economical cooking method if the oven is already in use.

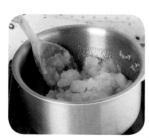

Stewing
Fruits such as apples and pears need to be softened by stewing them gently in a little water. The cooking liquid can then be added to the fruit when puréeing.

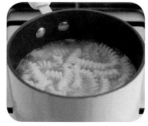

Boiling
Pasta, rice, and other grains need to be boiled in salt-free water, then drained before being mixed with other ingredients and served.

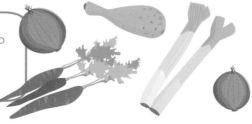

Meat and poultry need longer cooking times to become tender, so stewing with vegetables in water, or with salt-free stock, is the best cooking method.

2 Transfer cooked food to the equipment for puréeing

In the early weeks of weaning with purées, you need to make sure that your baby's food is the right consistency after cooking (see below) before serving it to your baby.

You can strain the cooked food through a sieve using a fork, or you might want to invest in some additional kitchen equipment to achieve a good purée.

Equipment

Some equipment combines several functions, while other items have just one or two uses. It's easy to be overwhelmed by the choice, so think about your requirements before purchasing. Do you want

something that produces food with different textures? Will you use it once your baby has passed the weaning stage? Is the equipment easy to clean and dishwasher friendly, and how much space does it take up?

A mouli (food grinder)
This utensil pushes food through a rotating grating disc to produce a fine consistency. In the UK, these are popular for potatoes, which become sticky in a blender or processor, but less commonly used for other foods.

A masher or ricer
A masher is good for making slightly lumpier textures, as is a ricer, which acts like a press that forces food through different-sized discs. Ricers have limited use, although are perfect for potatoes and root vegetables.

An electric hand blender
This makes great purées and can also be used to blend soups and get lumps out of sauces. Some come with attachments and other useful blades. Blenders with more than one speed can produce different textures.

Food processors, mini choppers, and blenders
Food processors can chop, slice, and purée; more compact mini choppers are also available. Models with different speeds help you control the texture of purées. A blender has fewer functions, but also purées well.

3 Blend until it is smooth

The consistency of first purées should be almost runny, similar to a non-set yogurt. If a purée is too thick, you can adjust the texture by adding your baby's usual milk or cooled boiled water. If it's too thin, add more of the food

or a spoonful of baby rice. Meat and poultry are usually introduced a bit later in the weaning process when your baby is starting to eat lumpier food, which is helpful as the fibres are more difficult to process finely.

Time to *eat*

You've cooked and cooled your baby's food, and you're ready to serve it up. There are a few items that are well worth buying or borrowing to help your baby's mealtimes go smoothly, allowing you and your baby to concentrate on the job at hand.

Serving your baby's food

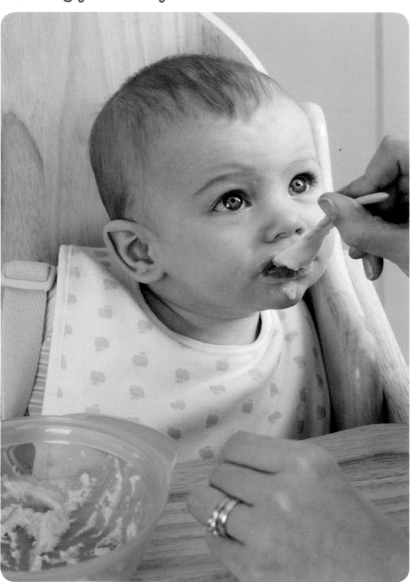

A secure feeding or high chair

A supportive high chair with straps ensures your baby is safely seated for feeding. When choosing one, think about your available space, whether the chair is easy to clean and portable (does it fold away when visiting friends or family?), and does it have a removable tray if you wish to draw your baby up to the table?

Bibs

These save on endless changes of outfit. Soft fabric bibs are comfy for younger babies, and all-in-one overall bibs are ideal for babies who are finger feeding. Pelican bibs have a collection tray at the bottom to catch dropped food.

Spoons

You need plenty of soft, long-handled, flexible plastic weaning spoons, which are more pleasant for your baby to put in her mouth than hard metal.

A lidded cup

This can be introduced from six months. Your baby can start to drink water or formula milk from a lidded cup, which helps with hand—eye coordination and learning to swallow.

Washing, sterilizing, and cleaning

- For babies under six months old, sterilize baby feeding spoons and bottles.
- After six months of age, wash your baby's food bowl and utensils in the dishwasher or in hot water and dry them with a clean tea towel.
- Clean your baby's high chair thoroughly after each meal, wiping away lodged food.
- Wash your baby's hands before she eats.

Make a mess!

As your baby grows, she will naturally start to explore food with her hands, which can be a messy business! It's tempting to mop her up as she goes along, but letting her interact with her food is an important part of learning. As she touches, squishes, and smears, she is finding out about texture, size, temperature, and shape. She is also developing her motor coordination as she finesses her grasp then attempts to transfer food from hand to mouth, exploration that will eventually lead to successful self-feeding with a spoon. Each new experience is exciting to your baby, and allowing her to explore food on her own terms means she is more likely to accept new foods and avoid being a fussy eater later on. Putting a splash mat or old newspapers under the high chair limits the chaos at ground level!

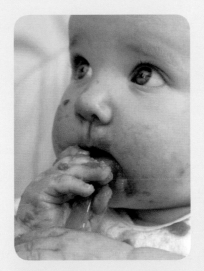
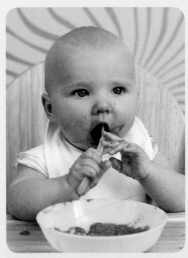
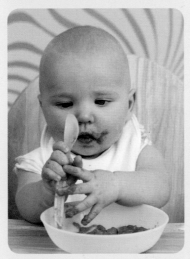
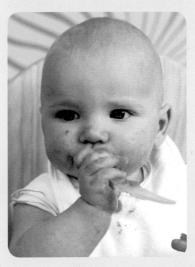

Is it an *allergy?*

Parents are often anxious about how and when to introduce foods that carry a higher risk of allergy to their baby's diet, and anxiety is fuelled by conflicting advice, with the latest research sometimes contradicting official guidelines. More children are developing adverse reactions to food, and if your child suffers a reaction this is alarming. Reassuringly, though, only a tiny proportion have serious or life-threatening reactions, and many children grow out of the most common allergies, to milk and eggs, by the age of five.

Allergy or intolerance?

Both of these mean that a food has caused an adverse reaction in the body, resulting in a "hypersensitivity" to the food. In an allergic reaction, the immune system reacts abnormally to a food, triggering the release of antibodies to the protein in the food, usually resulting in immediate symptoms. An intolerance doesn't involve the immune system and can be harder to spot as symptoms are slower to develop and can be linked to other childhood conditions.

Should my baby avoid gluten?

Wheat, rye, barley, and oats contain the protein gluten. Some people are genetically susceptible to gluten and cannot process it, which can result in coeliac disease, whereby the immune system treats gluten as a potential threat and attacks it, causing the gut to become sore and inflamed.

There's conflicting advice about when to introduce gluten. The UK government advises avoiding giving gluten-containing foods before six months. However, the European Food Safety Authority cites evidence that introducing it before six months (but not before 17 weeks) alongside breastfeeding may reduce the risk of developing coeliac disease, type 1 diabetes, and wheat allergy. The best advice may be to continue breastfeeding while you introduce wheat, rye, oats or barley, ensuring these aren't introduced before 17 weeks of age.

Recognizing a reaction

During an allergic reaction, your baby may have:

- A rash around the mouth, nose, and eyes
- Swelling of the lips, eyes, and face
- An itchy mouth and throat; the throat may be swollen
- A runny or blocked nose and watery eyes
- Sickness and diarrhoea

Symptoms of a food intolerance include:

- Diarrhoea or constipation, or blood or mucus in your baby's stools
- Colic
- Eczema
- Reflux

How do I respond?

If you suspect your baby has had a reaction to a food, it is very important to seek professional advice and not simply withdraw the food from your baby's diet indefinitely, as your baby could miss out on vital nutrients. Make a note of what your baby ate and the symptoms, then avoid giving the food again until you've spoken to your GP. Avoid, too, giving your baby similar foods to the one you suspect she reacted against. So if you think she reacted to cow's milk used in cooking, avoid other dairy products until you get advice. Depending on the severity of the reaction, your GP may refer your baby to an allergy clinic for further investigations.

Common culprits

The foods that most commonly cause allergic reactions are:

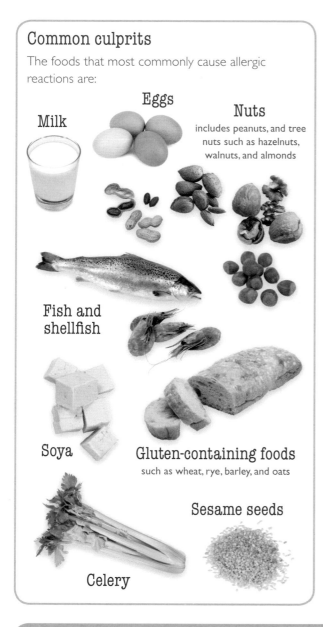

Milk

Eggs

Nuts
includes peanuts, and tree nuts such as hazelnuts, walnuts, and almonds

Fish and shellfish

Soya

Gluten-containing foods
such as wheat, rye, barley, and oats

Sesame seeds

Celery

Reducing the risks

There's conflicting evidence about whether it's best to delay introducing allergenic foods or introduce them early in the weaning process. Current advice is that potentially allergenic foods can be safely introduced once your baby is six months old. Foods only need to be introduced one at a time if your baby already has a diagnosed food allergy or you've been advised to do so.

Some families are genetically more predisposed to food allergies. If a close member of your baby's family has severe eczema, asthma, hayfever or allergies, she is at greater risk of developing an allergy than a baby whose family doesn't suffer. Also, if your baby has severe eczema, particularly if this started before three months, she has a higher risk of milk allergy. If her risk is higher, talk to your GP about introducing allergenic foods. Breastfeeding while weaning may offer some protection against developing allergies, so if your baby has a family history, you may be able to reduce her risk by continuing to breastfeed while weaning.

Living with an allergy

If your baby is diagnosed with an allergy, you will need to avoid the food as well as manufactured foods that could have traces of ingredients. These should be listed: the allergy clinic can also advise you on what names to look out for. A paediatric dietitian can advise you on how to ensure your baby doesn't miss out on important nutrients.

When visiting others, let them know in advance that your baby can't have certain products, and bring along your own food in case they forget about your baby's allergy.

A severe reaction (anaphylaxis) needing immediate medical attention includes:

- Wheezing, a cough, and breathing difficulties similar to an asthma attack
- Itchy skin or a red rash
- Swollen throat and tongue; may affect the voice
- A drop in blood pressure
- Confusion, dizziness, collapse, and unconsciousness

If you suspect your baby has anaphylaxis, call **999** immediately for an ambulance.

Weaning your *premature* baby

If your baby was born early (before 37 weeks), she may have missed out on some of the nutritional benefits of the last trimester of pregnancy, when babies build up stores of essential nutrients in the womb. In the first weeks and months, you may be advised to give your baby fortified formula milk or supplements if she is breastfed to provide vitamins and minerals, including iron, to ensure she grows and develops well. When you start to wean your baby, you will want to ensure that her nutritional needs continue to be met.

When should I wean my baby?

The actual date a premature baby is born on, rather than the expected due date you were given during pregnancy, is usually the date that is used to gauge when you should start to wean your baby onto solid foods. If your baby was very premature or very small at birth, then the medical team who cared for her in the first weeks and months should guide you on when to start weaning her onto solid foods. If your baby was only a few weeks premature and doesn't have any additional health problems, you will probably be advised to wean her around five to eight months from her actual birth date, and not to begin weaning before three months from her expected due date. As with all babies, she needs to show the signs that she is ready for solids (see p11). If you want further advice, talk to the medical team or your health visitor.

Will my baby take longer to wean?

Some premature babies develop conditions such as **reflux**. If this is the case, you will need specialist help from paediatric doctors, dietitians, and speech and language therapists to avoid nutritional and feeding problems.

Premature babies do sometimes take a little longer to learn to eat than babies born closer to their due date. Also, if your baby has had complex medical issues, for example a cleft palate, you may need the support of specialist dietitians and speech therapists when you start to wean, which can affect how long weaning takes. The menu planners in this book are still ideal for your baby, just be guided by her development. For example, if she is keen to eat, but slow to use her hands, you may need to cook and mash or chop some of the vegetable finger foods into her meal and spoon-feed for longer. She will catch up eventually, so try not to worry.

Does my baby need more calories?

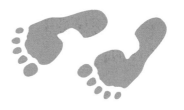

Each baby has their own individual nutritional requirements, whether or not they were premature. Health professionals will assess your baby by weighing and measuring her: if she is steadily gaining weight as expected, they will be happy that she is receiving sufficient calories. Once you start weaning, the advice is the same as for all babies, and you will need to ensure that your baby doesn't stay on purées of pure vegetables or fruits for too long as these are low in energy. If your baby has any developmental problems, this can mean that you need to introduce new textures more slowly, in which case you may want to mix fruit and vegetable purées with your baby's usual milk, or add a little baby rice to provide the calories your baby needs. If your baby had vitamin and mineral supplements after the birth, your health team will advise you on whether she needs to continue.

Does my baby need bigger portion sizes?

It's important not to try to help a smaller baby catch up on growth by encouraging her to eat excessively. Unless a health professional has advised you otherwise, your baby needs to be weaned in the same way as other babies with the same portion sizes.

Is my baby more susceptible to food allergies?

The digestive system of premature babies is not fully developed at birth, so it's natural to wonder if this means that your baby is at a greater risk than normal of developing food allergies. Reassuringly, several studies have shown that as long as you follow the guidelines for weaning and the advice of your health professionals this is not the case.

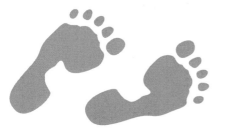

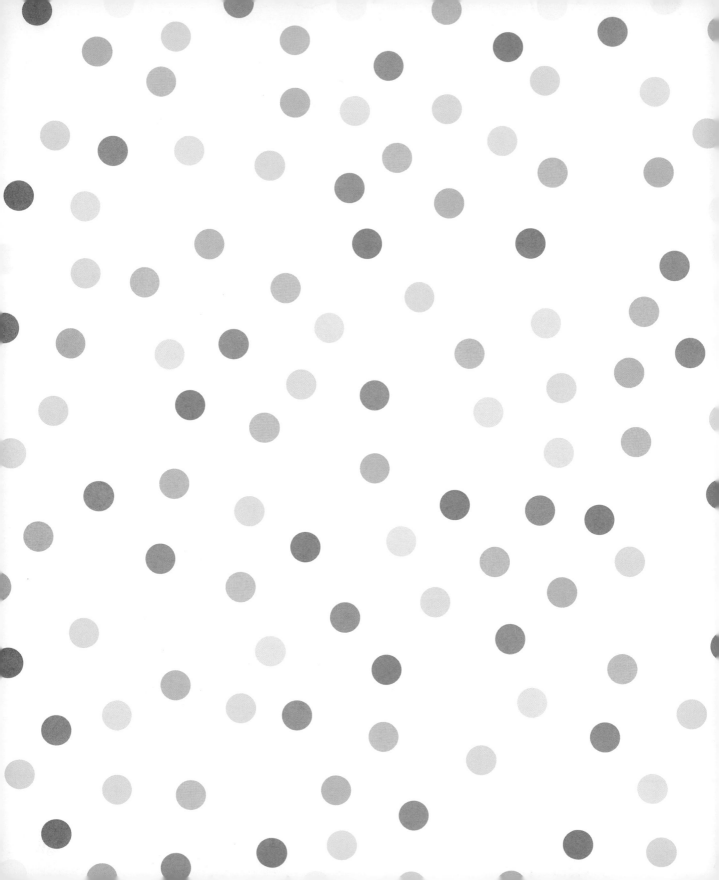

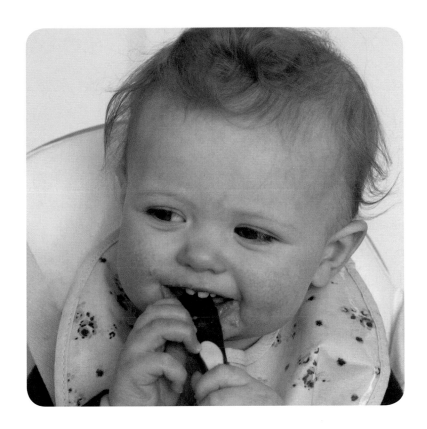

Day-by-day
planner

It's time to get started! In this section you'll find an introduction to each of the three stages of weaning, together with recipes for each age group and a menu plan for each day. The "menus" are no more complicated than one single taste at first, but the meals build up as the days and weeks go on.

How to use the
day-by-day planner

The day-by-day meal planners in this section cover the three stages of weaning: stage 1 up to seven months; stage 2 from seven to nine months, and stage 3 from nine to 12 months. The planners are designed to navigate you through each stage, providing a progression of textures and steadily introducing new tastes so that babies build up a repertoire of familiar foods and develop the ability to chew. The aim is that by the age of one, babies are eating foods from all the four main food groups and joining in with family meals.

Making the planner work for you

Stage 1 can be adapted depending on the age at which you start to wean your baby. There are eight weeks of planners here, so if you start at five months, you can follow it to the letter if you wish. Page 41 has advice on how to speed up this stage if you start closer to six months. If you think your baby may be ready to start solids before five months, consult your health visitor first; and never wean your baby before 17 weeks (see p11).

Each week provides a suggested daily menu for your baby appropriate for the weaning stage. So at the beginning of stage 1, there is just a single taste each day and by the end of this stage, your baby will be eating two simple meals a day. As your baby moves into stage 2, he will be having three regular meals each day. Each taste and meal is cross-referenced to the recipe pages. If you wish, you can follow the daily planners exactly, which will ensure that your baby receives a good balance of nutrients across the week. The quantities in most recipes make several meals, so you can freeze additional portions and use these when the recipe is repeated in a later week. From stage 2 onwards, variations are provided each week if you don't fancy making what's on the planner, or if your baby has an allergy or intolerance to a certain food in the planner. And if you wish, you can simply use the planners as a reference tool, for inspiration and guidance on the balance of foods to aim for.

From stage 2 onwards, there is a main meal each day and a lighter meal, as well as a breakfast suggestion. The main meal is usually listed as dinner, but this order doesn't need to be followed slavishly. If it's more convenient one day to have a main meal at lunchtime, then simply swap these around. Equally, many breakfast suggestions make good lunch options, or work well as puddings.

If you want to adapt the planner to suit the kind of day you're having, there are pages to help you. Pages 80–81 provide guidance on making the planner work when you're away from home, and pages 92–95 have other ideas for adapting the planners to suit your needs.

The planners in stage 1 follow the purée-based weaning route. If you wish to follow baby-led weaning, you will find that a variety of finger foods from the four main food groups are introduced around six months, which provide plenty of nutritional meal ideas. You can also offer some of the foods without puréeing if you wish.

If you are bringing up your baby as a vegetarian, you will find a good range of vegetarian recipes in the planners that you can use to form the basis of a varied diet for your baby. Page 76 lists the main sources of protein in a vegetarian diet, so you will need to ensure that your baby's daily diet includes adequate amounts of these.

Weaning twins

If you have twins, you may find that one baby is ready to wean earlier than the other, or that your twins progress at a different pace during the weaning process, perhaps one being happier to try new flavours, while the other is ready for lumps sooner. It's important to treat your twins as individuals and let each go at his own pace. You can adapt meals to suit each baby, perhaps removing a minced portion for one twin, then pulsing the rest of the meal for the other baby if he is not ready for this step up in texture. Batch cooking can also help you provide different tastes and textures for each one without having to cook up two different meals each time. As the aim of the weaning stages is for all babies to be joining in with family meals by 12 months, you should find that things even out as your twins get older.

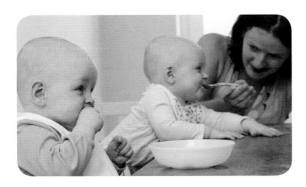

Thinking about allergies

With allergies on the rise in young children, there are certain foods that parents are currently advised to hold off on until after six months (see p41). The Stage 1 planners and recipes take this into account and avoid potentially allergenic foods under six months. (If you do start earlier than five months, make sure you avoid the foods listed on p41 until your baby reaches six months, repeating the early weeks as necessary.) From stage 2

onwards, recipes with peanuts are introduced. These usually appear as variations only in the planners so they're easy to avoid if you wish; the Creamy vegetarian mince (p126) appears in the main planner where peanuts appear as a variation to the main recipe, again making these easy to avoid. If you have a family history of allergies or feel unsure about introducing certain foods, talk to your doctor about the best approach.

Dealing with choking

It's natural for parents to worry about their baby choking when they start to eat solid food. Gagging and choking are hazards as your baby learns to coordinate the muscles needed for chewing with breathing. It's common for babies to gag sometimes when they start on solids: this is a natural reflex that happens when there's a risk of choking. Your baby is learning to regulate the amount of food he has in his mouth and to coordinate chewing and swallowing, so it's normal that he struggles sometimes. Try not to panic if your baby gags, as usually he will manage to move the food to the front of his mouth. This is also a valuable lesson for him in the importance of chewing. Choking occurs when the airway becomes completely obstructed and your baby is unable to breathe. The first aid box on page 220 explains what to do if your baby chokes, but there is no substitute for attending a first aid course or demonstration. Your local baby group may run one, or check information online from first aid societies such as The Red Cross.

You can reduce the risk of choking with simple measures such as removing skin on meats and fruits until your baby can chew more easily; halving foods such as grapes and cherry tomatoes that could block the windpipe if swallowed whole; and giving your baby lightly cooked foods before raw foods as he gets used to chewing. Always stay with your baby while he is eating so you can see if he is in trouble – a choking baby may not be able to cry or cough, so you can't rely on this to alert you.

Introducing *Stage 1*

This first phase of weaning, which usually starts at around five to six months and continues to around seven months, introduces your baby to the idea that food isn't always liquid, and, if you are following the puréeing route, that food comes on a spoon, from which your baby has to learn to move the food from the front of his mouth to the back to swallow it.

Progressing through the first stage

Your baby's first meals are mainly about experiencing new tastes and textures, as he will still be receiving everything he needs nutritionally from milk.

The menu planners and simple recipes guide you through the first weeks of weaning, suggesting ideal first foods for your baby, and ensuring that he learns to eat a wide range of nutritious foods. The planners for this stage cover a period of eight weeks, but can be extended or truncated if you wish to start earlier or later (see box, opposite).

What your baby eats now

For the first few months of your baby's life, milk is the most important food in his diet, providing all the nutrients and calories he needs. He should continue his usual milk feeds when you introduce solids.

- At around six months, milk still plays a key role, but no longer provides all the iron and zinc your baby needs, so he needs solid foods now, too.

- Simple single flavours are the best first foods for your baby; these are usually vegetables, fruits, and cereals such as rice or millet. Giving your baby one food at a time allows him to identify the individual flavours. This can be especially important with some bitter vegetables that are essential to a healthy, nutritious diet. Your baby needs to learn what broccoli or spinach tastes like, so don't be tempted to add sweet fruit or parsnip to his first taste of greens.

- After some single flavours, blends can be introduced.

- Meat, poultry, fish, and pulses, which provide minerals such as iron and zinc, should be introduced from around six months.

 New experiences

Studies show that it can take up to 10 tries for new foods to be accepted by babies, and research shows that it is easiest to introduce new or difficult flavours before seven months of age, so it's important to offer your baby vegetables repeatedly early on in the weaning process. Once your baby has become used to these first flavours, meat, poultry, fish, and pulses can be given towards the end of the first stage. Between five and seven months is a critical period when babies will accept difficult flavours such as green vegetables more readily than when these are left until after seven months.

Studies also show that babies who have only purées until nine months struggle to accept lumps. Make sure that early runny purées are followed up as soon as your baby can eat well from a spoon with thicker ones, then mashed foods. Finger foods, whether given as part of a mixed diet alongside purées or alone if you are doing baby-led weaning (see p21) are crucial in helping your baby learn to chew and cope with lumps.

STAGE 1 – at a glance

TEXTURE	During the first stage of weaning, the texture of your baby's food should progress from **runny purées** to **thicker purées**, then **mashed food**.	
INTRODUCE	By the end of stage 1, at around seven months, your baby should have tried: fruits · vegetables · cereals, including wheat · first meats · fish · pulses · dairy products · well-cooked eggs	
AVOID	Do not give processed meats such as sausages and ham, honey, liver, and whole nuts (see p19)	

Runny purée

Thicker purée

Mashed food

Starting early or late

If you start to give your baby first foods before he is six months old, you can move at a gentle pace through this first stage as milk will still be meeting his nutritional needs. We have given meal plans for eight weeks. If you introduce solids when your baby is five months old, you can follow the planner to the letter if you choose. If you wish to provide a bit more variety, you can try some of the other first tastes and blends recipes from the recipe pages.

If you wean your baby before six months, the common advice is to avoid giving him eggs, liver, nuts and seeds, fish and shellfish, dairy products, gluten-containing products such as wheat, and citrus fruits. The planner has been designed so your baby doesn't encounter these foods until after six months.

If you've waited until the recommended six months, your baby's need for nutrients and calories has increased, so it's important to progress through this stage quickly as fruit and vegetable purées are low in calories as well as iron and zinc. By six months of age, your baby shouldn't stay on vegetable and fruit purées alone for more than a week or two before moving quickly onto meat, poultry, fish, and pulses. This may mean not repeating some single flavours so often, especially fruits, which he is likely to favour anyway. The recipes often have common ingredients, so for example broccoli appears alone, then in combination with rice, then with rice and chicken, so if you wait until six months to wean, you could move from the simplest to more complex meals relatively quickly.

Your baby's *first meal*

Your baby's first meal can be quite an event as you decide which food you are going to start with, when is the best time to give it, and worry about whether or not your baby will like it. Your baby will pick up on your emotions, whether you are anxious or excited as his first mouthful approaches, and will be aware of how you react when that food goes in, and perhaps comes out again. So it's important to try to be as relaxed and positive as possible, which will be most likely if you're well prepared.

The first mouthful

Your baby's food is cooked and cooled and you're happy that it's the right consistency – a runny texture for first purées – so it's time to serve it up. Use the checklist here to help feeds go smoothly.

- Get your baby seated comfortably and securely in his high chair. If you are weaning before six months, your baby may not be able to sit upright easily in a high chair. You can hold him securely on your lap, or strap him into his bouncy chair if he has one.

- Put a bib on him – early feeding is messy, so this cuts down on endless changes of outfit.

- Use a soft-edged weaning spoon. If your baby is under six months old, this needs to be sterilized before use.

- Check the food is the right temperature before giving it to your baby. Test a little on the inside of your wrist – it should be neither hot nor cold.

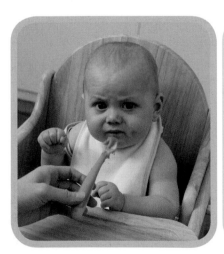

1 Bring the spoon to your baby's lips and let him open his mouth.

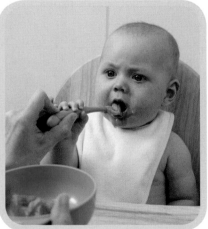

2 Gently move the spoon into his mouth so he can taste the food, letting him close his mouth around the spoon.

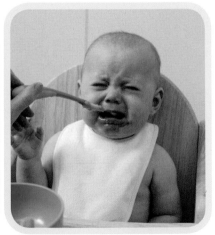

3 Some food may come out! Scoop it up and pop it back in.

If he likes it, try another spoon. If he's resistant, don't force it. Wait and try again with the next meal.

"Your baby's expression may not be quite what you expected. Wrinkling his nose doesn't necessarily mean he doesn't like a food. Try again and if he opens his mouth, you will know he is willing to give it a go. If he doesn't, just try another time."

Perfect timing

If you're feeling anxious about getting the timing right for your baby's first meal, bear in mind that he will be most responsive if he isn't too tired or too hungry. Your baby is used to satisfying his hunger quickly through drinking milk, so if he is very hungry, he won't cope well with the new experience of food on a spoon or tackling a finger food. Pick a time when he is alert and has had a small milk feed. Also choose a time that fits in with your day, too, as you need to be feeling calm and unrushed: it doesn't really matter whether this is breakfast time, lunchtime, or during the afternoon. Avoid later on in the day as you and your baby are more likely to be tired, and if he is unfortunate enough to react adversely to a food, you may miss any symptoms if he is put to bed soon after eating the food.

Good first purées

Your baby's first purées introduce him to a range of different vegetables, cereals, and fruits.

First breakfast cereals

Rice is often the first food given, and baby rice is fortified with vitamins and minerals. You can also try flaked millet.

A six-month-old baby can have cereals that contain grains such as wheat and barley, but look out for ones that are laden with sugar and/or salt.

First vegetables

Green and cruciferous vegetables are important in the diet as they contain iron and other essential nutrients.

broccoli • spinach • cauliflower • kale

Root vegetables often taste sweet, and orange root vegetables provide vitamin A. Potatoes, sweet potatoes, and yams are good sources of energy and useful for thickening purées.

carrot • parsnip • butternut squash • swede • turnip • pumpkin • sweet potato • yam • potato

Other vegetables that provide a mix of nutrients and tend to be liked by babies include:

peas • sweetcorn

First fruits

Different-coloured fruits provide a range of vitamins and phytonutrients, which are naturally occurring substances that help protect the body from disease.

apple • pear • banana • apricot • avocado • mango • peach • blueberry

How much is *enough?*

Now that your baby is starting to eat solid food, you may be concerned about just how much food he needs. In fact, he has a built-in mechanism to help him know when he is full – you simply need to learn to read the signs that he has had enough. As a rough guide, in the first few days he will probably only have a few mouthfuls, the equivalent of a teaspoon or two, at a time. The quantity will increase as he learns how to swallow food and starts to enjoy different flavours, building up to two or more tablespoons per meal as your baby moves into the second stage of weaning (see p76).

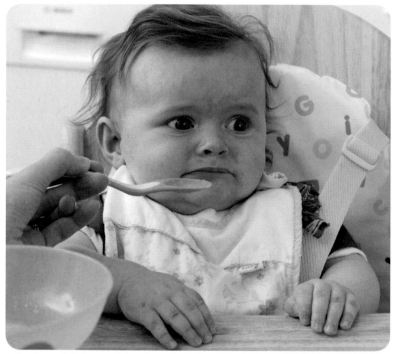

Read your baby's cues. If that final mouthful is refused, she's telling you she's full.

Reading the signs

There are several signs to look out for to help you recognize when your baby has eaten enough:

- He may turn his head to one side to avoid another spoonful.

- He may refuse to open his mouth after he has eaten a few mouthfuls.

- He may spit food out. In the early stages, he may do this anyway if he hasn't lost his extrusion reflex, which causes him to push food to the front of his mouth. If this is the case, he may not be ready to wean and you might need to wait another week or two before trying again, until he is able to move the food from the front to the back of his mouth.

Following your baby's lead

Researchers have been looking at how to prevent young children from becoming overweight. Studies suggest that encouraging a baby to have more than he naturally eats or coercing him to clear his plate can have an adverse affect on his ability to self-regulate his intake of food. However, other research shows that being too concerned about overfeeding and restricting your child's intake of food is not helpful either. It can be tricky for parents to find the right balance. Try to be guided by your baby, watching for cues that he is full (see above) and not pressurizing him to eat more if he seems reluctant.

Your baby's milk feeds

Towards the end of stage one, your baby will be having two meals a day, including breakfast. However, these will consist of just a few spoonfuls of purée or cereal, so he will still be having his usual quantity of milk, around four to five breastfeeds, or approximately 600ml (1 pint) formula each day.

As your baby moves through the weaning process, the quantity of milk will drop off gradually. If you continue breastfeeding, your baby will usually naturally reduce the amount of milk he takes, allowing your breasts to adjust and in turn reduce the amount of milk they produce. If you wish to wean your baby off the breast and onto formula, you will need to plan this more carefully. The advice is to do this slowly, if possible. This is more reassuring for your baby; he is used to the comfort of breastfeeding and is likely to become distressed if this is removed too quickly. Moving gradually from breast to bottle also reduces the risk of your breasts becoming uncomfortably engorged. Ideally, do this over a period of weeks, each week replacing one breastfeed in the day with a bottle feed.

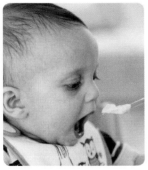 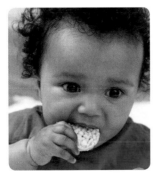 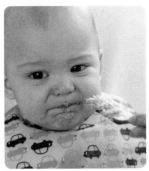 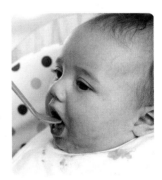

Your baby's enthusiasm for his food will be evident. Go at his pace, taking it slowly if he's a bit more cautious.

Portion sizes

The portions shown below are suitable for babies who have accepted first tastes.
All babies vary in the amount they eat, and as they grow more is eaten at each meal.

FOOD GROUP	TYPICAL MEAL	TYPICAL AMOUNT FOR UP TO 7 MONTHS OLD
Vegetables and fruits given singly	First tastes – any meal	5 teaspoons per meal
Infant cereal or potato mixed with milk	Breakfast	1–5 teaspoons of cereal/potato mixed with 4–10 teaspoons milk
Meat, poultry, fish, eggs or pulses mixed with vegetables	Lunch or dinner	5 teaspoons per meal
Milk – formula or breast milk	Throughout the day	Minimum 600ml (1 pint) formula milk or 4–5 breastfeeds
Dairy foods alone or mixed with fruit	Dessert or breakfast	5 teaspoons per meal
High-fat and high-sugar foods	Not suitable	Not suitable

Your *thirsty* baby

Throughout the first year, your baby will continue to rely on breast or formula milk as a major source of energy and some nutrients. However, as he grows he will also need additional fluids for growth and to replace fluids lost in urine, faeces, and sweating. Water is readily absorbed and used by the body and, other than milk, is the best drink for babies. Tap water is preferable as some mineral waters contain too much sodium or sulphate. As he can't express his need for fluids, you will need to offer drinks with meals in addition to his daily milk.

How much should my baby drink?

Before six months of age, bottlefed babies often need additional water to avoid constipation, while exclusively breastfed babies don't need extra water. Tap water is best, and under six months, this should be boiled first then cooled before giving it to your baby. Once you introduce solids, your baby's need for water increases, whether he's breast- or bottlefed. A baby between six and 12 months of age needs to drink around one litre of fluid a day, which will be supplied in part by breast or formula milk, and the balance from other drinks and foods. There's no need to boil and cool water first after six months. You don't need to measure out water for your baby in addition to his milk, but offer him a drink with his meals so that he can self-regulate the amount he needs. If he is unwell, he may need additional fluids, especially if he goes off his milk feeds.

It's important for your baby to learn how to control his appetite and to recognize the difference between hunger and thirst. If you give him too many drinks, with the exception of water, between meals, he may struggle to learn these innate cues.

Cups and bottles

Once your baby is getting used to eating solids, it's time to ditch bottles and teats and introduce lidded beakers with spouts. This is because he needs to learn to sip rather than suck, and fluids, especially if they are sweetened, need to be in the mouth for as short a time as possible to minimize the risk of damage to his emerging teeth. You can buy fast-flow spouts for bottles to start your baby with at six months, but, as soon as possible, and certainly by 12 months, he should be drinking all bottled drinks, including formula milk, from a cup with or without a lid.

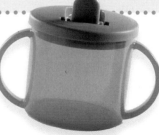

Cups with lids and spouts

Cups, or beakers, with lids, spouts, and easy-to-hold handles are ideal first cups for your baby, helping to ease the transition from bottle to cup. Cups with spouts that flip up are easy flow, and non-spill when the spout is down; non-flip spouts require more sucking.

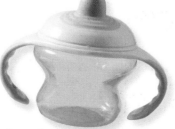

What about juice and flavoured drinks?

Even unsweetened fruit juices contain naturally present sugars, which is why milk and water are the best drinks for your baby. There are three main reasons to avoid sweetened drinks:

• Sweetened fluids can damage your baby's teeth.

• Your baby may develop a preference for sweetened foods and drinks.

• It is easy to over-consume sweetened drinks and this can lead to your baby being overweight.

If you are bringing up your baby as a vegetarian, you can offer him unsweetened fruit juice, diluted one part juice to 10 parts water, at mealtimes, as the vitamin C in the juice helps iron absorption from plant-based foods. Otherwise it's best to offer plain water at mealtimes.

If you do want to give your baby fruit juice, make sure it is unsweetened, diluted, and offer it only at mealtimes in a beaker, not a bottle with a teat, so it can be quickly sipped. Don't give your baby drinks other than milk or water between meals. Any other drinks should definitely be avoided. Fruit squashes have added sugar, and low-sugar or diet squashes contain sweeteners that are not suitable for babies. Flavoured milks are high in sugar, and fizzy drinks aren't suitable for babies or young children as they are acidic and damage teeth. Sweetened herbal drinks, or drinks marketed as baby cordials or squashes aren't suitable for babies, and don't be tempted to give even diluted tea or coffee as these contain caffeine and tannin, which interfere with iron absorption.

Your baby's milk

If you've been breastfeeding and want to move to formula, which type is best for your baby? And if your baby has been on formula, should you change to a different type as he grows?

• Infant formula is suitable for babies up to and beyond one year.

• Follow-on formula is an iron-fortified formula that is suitable from six months of age. If your baby is receiving all his iron needs from his diet, this shouldn't be necessary.

• Growing-up milk is an enriched formula suitable only from one year.

• Soya formula should only be used on the advice of a health professional as this can be allergenic and there are health concerns about the phyto-oestrogens (plant hormones) it contains. Soya formula also contains sugars that can damage teeth.

Other milks:

• Cow's milk isn't suitable as a drink until one year. At 12 months, full-fat cow's milk can be introduced as a drink. Semi-skimmed milk can be introduced from two years of age if your toddler is growing well and has a healthy and varied diet.

• Soya milk is not suitable for children under the age of two as it is too low in iron, fat, and calories. Occasionally, a toddler may be advised to use a special toddler soya milk on medical grounds.

• Rice or nut milks aren't suitable for children under the age of five as they are nutritionally inadequate.

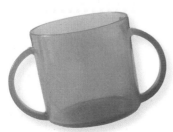

Open cup with handles

By one year, possibly earlier, encourage your baby to drink from a cup without a lid.

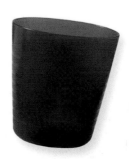

Open cup

As your child grows and his dexterity increases, he will manage a confident hold on a plastic cup without handles.

Setting up *good habits*

Your baby probably developed his taste buds before you even knew you were pregnant, and they matured about 15 weeks after conception, just before the development of his taste receptors. Babies in the womb swallow amniotic fluid constantly, so by the time your baby was born, he would have experienced plenty of flavours from the foods you ate while you were pregnant.

Shaping your baby's tastes

Your baby learns from watching you, and he will mimic your behaviour, whether you like it or not! So he is much more likely to learn to love eating vegetables if he sees you and your partner eating and enjoying them. If, on the other hand, he senses that broccoli is a necessary evil that he is forced to eat but you won't countenance, you will have some difficulties ahead.

Eating together is much more fun for your baby than eating alone, so whenever you can, eat with him. If possible, let him watch you prepare his meal, showing him what it contains. It is good for him to learn, for example, what a carrot looks like, so as he progresses from purées to mashed then chopped carrots, he is not surprised when it appears in a different form. Baby food is, after all, real food provided in an appropriate texture.

Towards the end of the first stage, you can start to introduce your baby to a range of soft finger foods, or you may start him off on finger foods at six months if you choose to follow baby-led weaning. Encouraging your baby to move towards more independent eating helps him to embrace new foods as he learns to eat on his own terms. Likewise, if your baby grabs the spoon while you feed him, let him have a go himself. If you're worried that not much of the food is making it to his mouth, you could use two spoons, one for him to hold and one that you keep to pop some food into his mouth between his attempts. Try not to get frustrated if this slows down mealtimes a little; letting him have a go helps him to feel involved and interested in his food, so by the time he reaches his first birthday, he should be happy and relaxed joining in with family meals.

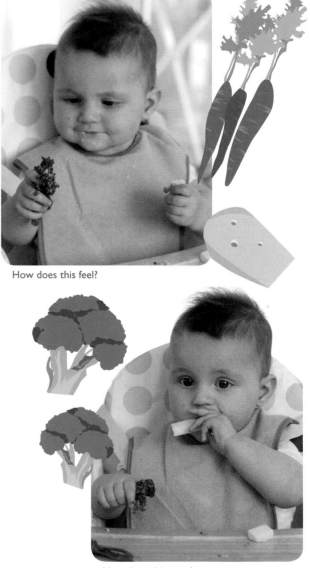

How does this feel?

How does this taste?

My baby won't eat!

It's not uncommon for babies to go off food when they had previously been feeding well, or to resist the transition to solids. There are many reasons why babies refuse food; understanding why can help you avoid worrying about your baby's wellbeing.

- Your baby may not feel like eating if he's unwell, especially if it's early on in the weaning process when he will be comforted by the familiarity of milk rather than the newness of solids. Teething babies can also go off food if their gums hurt and they feel out of sorts. Try not to worry; simply try food again once he's feeling better, maybe starting with one of the foods that he clearly likes first.

- If your baby resists a food when first introduced, check that he is developmentally ready for solids (see p11). If he doesn't show these signs, you might need to hold off on solids for a while longer.

- Your baby may not feel like eating if he is already full of milk. Be guided by his appetite, and don't encourage him to finish bottles if he's unwilling.

Made with love

You may have spent a lot of time preparing your baby's food. If this doesn't always get eaten – perhaps your baby isn't keen on a flavour or isn't very hungry – you may question whether it's worth the effort. So what are the advantages of home-made food, and are there times when commercial foods are fine for your baby?

Pros of home-made food

- It's important for your baby to accept new textures. Home-made food has more variations in texture, and even the same dish won't be the same each time, so your baby learns it's okay when a dish feels different.

- Your baby will have experienced some flavours while in the womb and breastfeeding, so he's likely to be receptive to these when he encounters them again.

- If properly prepared and cooked, home-made food can contain more vitamin C and B group vitamins than pouches or jars of foods.

- Your baby can see foods being made so is less likely to be wary of ingredients.

- Home-made food is more cost-effective, especially if making in bulk for freezing.

Pros of commercial baby foods

- If the family diet is poor, using some commercial foods ensures some good nutrients for your baby.

- Strictly regulated sourcing means ingredients are sometimes better than ones used at home.

- Pouches and jars are convenient for travelling and as emergency storecupboard food.

- If parents have dietary restrictions, bought baby food can provide foods they can't eat.

- Some family foods, such as those containing salt, aren't suitable for babies.

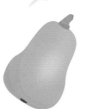

day-by-day meal planner
Week 1

If you've waited until six months to begin weaning, you can skip week one, moving straight to week two with two tastes each day.

Day 1
First taste
Baby rice p58

Day 2
First taste
Carrot p58

Day 3
First taste
Carrot p58

Day 4
First taste
Broccoli p58

Day 5
First taste
Broccoli p58

Day 6
First taste
Pear p59

Day 7
First taste
Pear p59

How much milk?
Your baby needs to continue breastfeeding or having the same amount of infant formula each day.

You don't need to follow the plan slavishly, but do try to introduce broccoli, cauliflower, and spinach in the first two weeks.

day-by-day meal planner
Week 2

Day 1
First taste
Butternut squash p59

Second taste
Pear p59

Day 2
First taste
Butternut squash p59

Second taste
Mango p59

Day 7
First taste
Cauliflower p60

Second taste
Blueberry p60

Day 6
First taste
Cauliflower p60

Second taste
Mango p59

Day 3
First taste
Apple p59

Second taste
Broccoli p58

How much milk?
Your baby needs to continue breastfeeding or having the same amount of infant formula each day.

Day 5
First taste
Spinach p59

Second taste
Banana p59

Day 4
First taste
Spinach p59

Second taste
Apple p59

day-by-day meal planner
Week 3

If you've waited until six months to begin weaning, move onto blends and firmer textures quickly, minimizing the number of blends you use, and moving quickly onto meals. Or skip weeks one, three, and seven.

Day 1
Breakfast
Banana p59

Second meal
Pea p60

Day 2
Breakfast
Apricot p60

Second meal
Pea p60

Day 3
Breakfast
Apple p59

Second meal
Carrot and squash p63

Day 4
Breakfast
Plum and apple p63

Second meal
Carrot and squash p63

Day 5
Breakfast
Mango p59

Second meal
Cauliflower and sweet potato p63

Day 6
Breakfast
Avocado p61

Second meal
Cauliflower and sweet potato p63

Day 7
Breakfast
Millet and banana porridge p68

Second meal
Broccoli, pea, and potato p65

How much milk?
Your baby needs to continue breastfeeding or having the same amount of infant formula each day.

day-by-day meal planner
Week

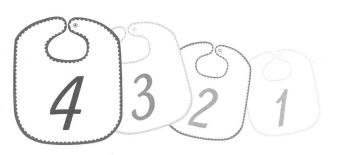

4 3 2 1

Day 1
Breakfast
Mango p59

Second meal
Courgette, spinach, and tomato p64

Day 7
Breakfast
Apricot porridge p68

Second meal
Broccoli, pea, and potato p65

Day 2
Breakfast
Apple and yogurt p67

Second meal
Courgette, spinach, and tomato p64

Day 6
Breakfast
Apple and yogurt p67

Second meal
Broccoli, pea, and potato p65

How much milk?
Your baby needs to continue breastfeeding or having the same amount of infant formula each day.

Day 3
Breakfast
Peach p61 or pear p59

Second meal
Carrot, leek, and potato p64

Day 5
Breakfast
Mango p59 or pear p59

Second meal
Parsnip and sweet potato p65

Day 4
Breakfast
Yogurt with cinnamon and pear p67

Second meal
Carrot, leek, and potato p64

day-by-day meal planner
Week 5 4 3

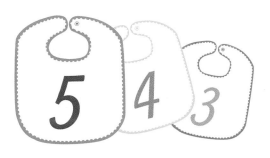

Don't forget to offer your baby water with his meals (see p46).

Day 1
Breakfast
Apricot and pear p66

Second meal
Sweetcorn, squash, and tomato p65

Day 2
Breakfast
Banana oat porridge p68

Second meal
Beef, carrot, and potato p74

Day 3
Breakfast
Wheat biscuit with milk p70

Second meal
Sweetcorn, squash, and tomato p65

Day 4
Breakfast
Apple and yogurt p67

Second meal
Beef, carrot, and potato p74

Day 5
Breakfast
Banana slices and yogurt p67

Second meal
Cauliflower, cheese, and potato p71

Day 6
Breakfast
Plum and yogurt p67

Second meal
Cauliflower, cheese, and potato p71

Day 7
Breakfast
Apricot porridge p68

Second meal
Salmon and sweet potato p72

How much milk?
Your baby needs to continue breastfeeding or having the same amount of infant formula each day.

day-by-day meal planner
Week 6

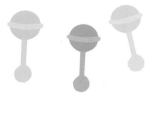
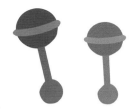

Day 1
Breakfast
Orchard fruits
breakfast p70

Second meal
Salmon and
sweet potato p72

Day 2
Breakfast
Blueberry
and yogurt p67

Second meal
Lamb and apricots
with rice p75

Day 7
Breakfast
Apple and yogurt p67

Second meal
Butterbean, parsnip, and
sweet potato p73

Day 3
Breakfast
Apricot and pear,
buttered toast p69

Second meal
Lamb and apricots
with rice p75

Day 6
Breakfast
Orchard fruits
breakfast p70

Second meal
Avocado and banana p66

How much milk?
You may notice your baby
wants a little less of his milk
feed, but continue as you
have been doing.

Day 5
Breakfast
Wheat biscuit
with milk p70

Second meal
Potato, spinach,
and ricotta p71

Day 4
Breakfast
Mango and yogurt p67

Second meal
Potato, spinach,
and ricotta p71

day-by-day meal planner Week 7

If you've waited until six months to begin weaning, you can skip weeks one, three, and seven.

Day 1
Breakfast
Yogurt with cinnamon and pear p67

Second meal
Lentil, tomato, and coriander dhal p73

Soft pear slices

Day 2
Breakfast
Apricot porridge p68

Second meal
Lentil, tomato, and coriander dhal p73

Plum and apple p63

Day 7
Breakfast
Orchard fruits breakfast p70 and buttered toast p69

Second meal
Chicken and broccoli with rice p74

Apricot and yogurt p67

How much milk?
You may notice your baby wants a little less of his milk feed, but continue as you have been doing.

Day 3
Breakfast
Plum and yogurt p67

Second meal
Potato, spinach, and ricotta p71

Banana slices

Day 6
Breakfast
Wheat biscuit with milk and banana slices p70

Second meal
Cod, pea, and potato p72

Plum and apple p63

Day 5
Breakfast
Banana oat or millet porridge p68

Second meal
Cod, pea, and potato p72

Fromage frais with apricot purée p70

Day 4
Breakfast
Yogurt, banana slices, and buttered toast p69

Second meal
Lamb and apricots p75

Blueberry purée p60 with rice

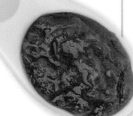

day-by-day meal planner
Week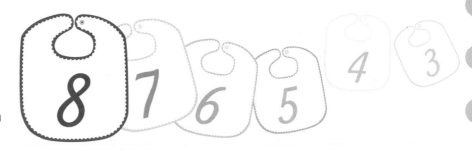

Day 1
Breakfast
Hard-boiled egg and buttered toast p69

Second meal
Chicken and broccoli with rice p74

Banana slices or purée

Day 2
Breakfast
Fromage frais with blueberry purée p70

Second meal
Salmon and sweet potato p72

Apple and mango or soft fruit pieces

Day 3
Breakfast
Sliced banana and yogurt p67

Second meal
Salmon and sweet potato p72

Fromage frais with apricot purée p70

Day 4
Breakfast
Yogurt with cinnamon and pear p67

Second meal
Beef, carrot, and potato p74

Apple purée p59

Day 5
Breakfast
Apricot porridge p68 and buttered toast p69

Second meal
Beef, carrot, and potato p74

Peach slices with yogurt p67

Day 6
Breakfast
Wheat biscuit with milk and soft pear or mango pieces p70

Second meal
Butterbean, parsnip, and sweet potato p73

Blueberry purée with yogurt p67

Day 7
Breakfast
Hard-boiled egg and buttered toast p69

Second meal
Butterbean, parsnip, and sweet potato p73

Banana and pear slices

How much milk?
You may notice your baby wants a little less of his milk feed, but continue as you have been doing.

Single *tastes*

The first tastes your baby tries give him the chance to try small amounts of different foods and learn that food comes in forms other than liquid. There are plenty of purées here to try over the first couple of weeks. Some, such as banana, avocado or baby rice are made up fresh each time, while others can be made in batches to freeze. Starting off with single flavours helps your baby distinguish different foods. Try to give vegetables more often than fruit in the first week or two so your baby doesn't develop a taste for sweet foods. As your baby gets used to solids, thicken purées by using less water or milk, or by adding a little baby rice or mashed potato. The portion sizes here are suitable for stage 1 weaning (see pp44–45).

Freezing your baby's food

It's best to cook foods before freezing them. Where a purée or meal is suitable for freezing, after cooking remove a portion to eat straightaway, then cool the remainder before freezing in a container (see p.27) marked with the date and food. Use all purées within six months, defrosting them in a fridge set at less than 4°C (39.2°F).

Baby rice

This easily dissolvable vitamin-fortified powder is a popular first food, letting your baby adjust to a new texture while enjoying the familiar flavour of milk. Baby rice can also be used to thicken purées as your baby progresses through the first stage of weaning.

  1 portion

ingredients
Your **baby's usual milk**
Baby rice

method
1 Follow the instructions on the packet: usually 1 teaspoon (2g) baby rice is used for every tablespoon (15ml) of milk.

Carrot

Carrots are a wonderful source of vitamin A, and their sweet taste makes them a popular vegetable with babies and toddlers alike.

 7–8 mins   4–5 portions

ingredients
1 large **carrot**
60ml (2fl oz) cooled boiled **water**, or your **baby's usual milk**

method
1 Peel the carrot and trim off the top and bottom. Cut into 1cm (½in) cubes or slice thinly.

2 Steam for 7–8 minutes, or until tender.

3 Cool slightly, then purée with the water or milk.

Broccoli

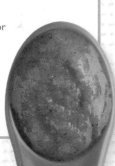

This is high in vitamins A and C and also provides some iron; it's worth introducing this purée early as broccoli is an important staple of a healthy diet.

 8–10 mins

 8–10 portions

ingredients
150g (5½oz) **broccoli** florets, washed
120ml (4floz) cooled boiled **water**, or your **baby's usual milk**

method
1 Steam the broccoli for 8–10 minutes until tender.

2 Cool slightly, then purée with the water or milk.

Pear

Pears are a classic first weaning food as they don't cause allergic reactions. Use ripe pears that are not too grainy, such as comice or conference.

 5–6 mins

6-8... 8–10 portions

ingredients
2 medium ripe **pears**
1tsp or so cooled boiled **water**, or **your baby's usual milk**, if required

method
1 Peel the pears, quarter, and remove the cores. Dice and steam for 5–6 minutes.

2 Cool slightly, then purée the pears with the water or milk if required.

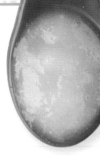

Squash

Butternut or other squashes, such as pumpkin or acorn squash, purée easily and have protective vitamin A. Use ready-prepared fresh or frozen squash if you want a small quantity.

 10–12 mins

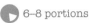 6–8 portions

ingredients
150g (5½oz) **butternut squash**
90ml (3fl oz) cooled boiled **water**, or your **baby's usual milk**

method
1 Peel the squash and cut into cubes, around 1–2cm (½–¾in) in size.

2 Steam for 10–12 minutes or until tender.

3 Cool slightly; purée with water or milk.

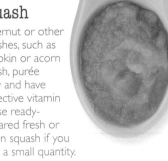

Mango

Rich in vitamin C, mangoes make a tasty purée. The fruit should yield slightly when pressed. Use unsweetened canned mango purée when fresh is out of season.

  2 portions

ingredients
80–100g (3–3½oz) or about one quarter, fresh ripe **mango**, cut into cubes

method
1 Purée the mango cubes until smooth.

2 Use half immediately, then refrigerate the rest in an airtight container for 24 hours.

* Variation: *Mix with strawberry purée and/or yogurt for a simple and delicious dessert or breakfast.*

Apple

Universally enjoyed, this is often one of the first fruits a baby eats. Any eating apple will do, but a sweet, softer flesh purées more easily than a crisp apple.

 7–9 mins

 6–8 portions

ingredients
2 medium eating **apples**
75ml (2½fl oz) cooled boiled **water** or **your baby's usual milk**

method
1 Peel and core the apples. Cut into quarters, then cut each quarter into smaller pieces, about 1cm (½in) in size.

2 Steam for 7–9 minutes until soft. Remove from the heat.

3 Cool slightly then purée the apple with the water or milk.

Spinach

Providing vitamins A, C, and K, and iron, spinach has great nutritional credentials. You can add some of your baby's milk to sweeten it a little.

 5–6 mins

 6–7 portions

ingredients
150g (5½oz) fresh **spinach leaves**
30ml (1fl oz) cooled boiled **water** or your **baby's usual milk**, if needed

method
1 Wash the leaves. Drain in a colander, then place in a large lidded saucepan.

2 Bring to the boil, then simmer and cook until the leaves wilt.

3 Cool slightly, then purée, adding water or milk, if required.

* Tip: *Add to other foods once accepted.*

Banana

Possibly an all time baby favourite, banana is a very easy purée to make. With no preparation or cooking required, all you need is a fork, plate, and banana for an instant meal on the move.

  1 portion

ingredients
½ small ripe **banana**

method
1 Peel the banana and chop or slice roughly.

2 Using a fork, mash until the banana becomes a smooth purée. Use immediately.

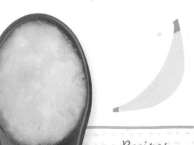

Cauliflower

This is a good source of vitamin C and the B vitamin folate. Both nutrients are reduced during cooking, so steam and cool rapidly to preserve as many nutrients as possible.

8–10 mins

6–8 portions

ingredients

150g (5½oz) **cauliflower** florets, washed

90ml (3fl oz) cooled boiled **water** or your **baby's usual milk**

method

1 Steam the cauliflower florets for 8–10 minutes, or until tender.

2 Cool slightly, then purée with the water or milk.

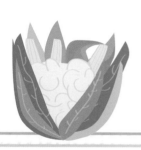

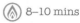
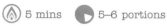

Blueberry

Blueberries purée easily, but because of their seeds and skin, they don't become absolutely smooth, so you may want to wait to make this one until your baby has become accustomed to eating from a spoon. Add to yogurt or a little baby rice to make a simple dessert or breakfast.

5 mins   5–6 portions

ingredients

100g (3½oz) **blueberries**
2 tbsp **water**

method

1 Wash the blueberries and place in a small saucepan with the water.

2 Heat for 3–4 minutes, breaking up the berries with a wooden spoon.

3 When the berries have softened, remove from the heat and cool slightly. Blend with the liquid until you have a purée.

* Variation: *If you want a thicker purée, add 2 teaspoons of baby rice, stirring well until it is mixed thoroughly.*

Pea

Peas are sweet and full of vitamin C. However, they can be difficult to purée completely finely, so it's probably best to hold back on giving your baby this purée until first tastes are well established. Use frozen petit pois rather than garden peas as they are less fibrous and easier to purée.

5–6 mins   4–6 portions

ingredients

100g (3½oz) frozen **petit pois**

75ml (2½fl oz) cooled boiled **water** or your **baby's usual milk**

method

1 Steam the peas for 5–6 minutes until very tender.

2 Cool slightly, then purée with the water or milk.

Apricot

Fresh apricots have a short season only, so at other times of the year make this firm baby favourite using dried apricots, or simply purée canned apricots in fruit juice. This purée is great to pop into some yogurt or fromage frais for a simple breakfast or dessert.

10–15 mins   8–10 portions

ingredients

100g (3½oz) ready-to-eat **apricots**

250ml (9fl oz) **water**

method

1 Place the apricots in a small saucepan and pour over the water.

2 Cover with a lid and bring to the boil, then reduce the heat, and simmer until the apricots are soft.

3 Cool slightly and purée with the cooking liquid until runny, adding more cooled boiled water if required.

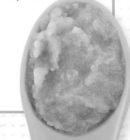

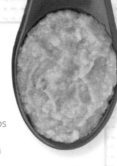

Avocado

These provide energy from healthy fats as well as vitamin E, and are an enjoyable creamy first food. All you need to prepare them is a sharp knife and a fork for mashing, making avocados an easily portable meal for babies. Lemon or lime juice prevents the flesh from browning, but isn't essential.

  1 portion

ingredients

¼ ripe **avocado**

1 tsp **lemon** or **lime juice**, optional

method

1 Cut the avocado flesh into cubes and sprinkle over the juice, if using.

2 Mash with a fork until you have a smooth, creamy purée, and use immediately.

✱ **Variation:** Mix avocado and banana for a popular baby meal (see p.66).

Peach

Seasonal peaches or nectarines make a runny purée, suitable from early on. Like most soft fruit they are best fresh. As soon as your baby can hold foods, you can give fingers of skinned peach.

  1 portion

ingredients

1 small or ½ medium ripe **peach** or **nectarine**

method

1 Using a sharp knife, remove the skin, and stone the peach or nectarine (see tip, below).

2 Cut the flesh into chunks, purée until smooth, and use immediately.

✱ **Tip:** To remove the skin, fill a small bowl with boiling water and place the fruit in the bowl for 1 minute. Remove with a slotted spoon, and using a small sharp knife, peel away the skin.

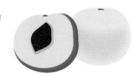

Plum

These are a good source of vitamin A. Choose ripe fruit that yields a little when gently pressed.

 10–12 mins 5–6 portions

ingredients

2 medium **plums**, washed and stoned, cut into quarters

100ml (3½fl oz) **water**

method

1 Place the plums and water in a saucepan and bring to the boil.

2 Reduce the heat, cover, and simmer until the fruit is tender.

3 Cool slightly before puréeing.

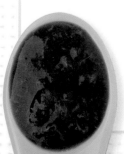

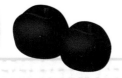

Swede

This is an inexpensive root vegetable that has a slight sweetness, making it popular with babies.

 7–8 mins 6–8 portions

ingredients

160g (5¾oz) or one small piece of **swede**, peeled and cut into 5mm (¼in) cubes

90ml (3fl oz) cooled boiled **water** or your **baby's usual milk**

method

1 Steam the swede for 7–8 minutes or until tender.

2 Cool slightly, then purée with the water or milk.

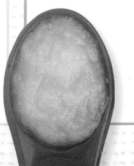

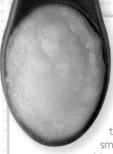

Parsnip

With a mild, sweet flavour and creamy texture, parsnips are a favourite first vegetable, and this purée is ideal for adding to other vegetable, meat, or poultry purées in the early weeks of weaning. Choose smaller parsnips, as large ones tend to be a bit woody in the centre so purée less well.

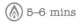 5–6 mins   6–8 portions

ingredients

1 medium or 2 small **parsnips**

90ml (3fl oz) cooled boiled **water**, or your **baby's usual milk**

method

1 Peel the parsnip and trim off the top and bottom. Slice thinly, discarding any particularly woody parts. Steam for 5–6 minutes, or until tender.

2 Cool slightly, then purée with the water or milk.

Sweetcorn

Once your baby has become used to a few flavours and you are making less runny purées, try sweetcorn. Like peas, sweetcorn is more fibrous than some vegetables and the smoothness of your purée will depend on the efficiency of your processor or blender. Frozen sweetcorn can be used to make a simple, cost effective purée. Sweetcorn provides essential vitamin B3 (niacin).

 3–5 mins   4–6 portions   ❄

ingredients

100g (3½oz) frozen **sweetcorn**

60ml (2fl oz) cooled boiled **water**, or your **baby's usual milk**

method

1 Steam the sweetcorn for 3–5 minutes until tender.

2 Cool slightly, then purée with the water or milk.

Sweet potato

Unlike ordinary potatoes, sweet potatoes purée easily, making them a great baby food. They also provide generous amounts of vitamin A.

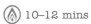 10–12 mins   6–8 portions

ingredients

150g (5½oz) or 1 small **sweet potato**

120ml (4fl oz) cooled boiled **water** or your **baby's usual milk**

method

1 Peel the sweet potato and cut into 1cm (½in) cubes. Steam for 10–12 minutes until soft.

2 Cool slightly, then purée with the water or milk.

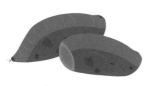
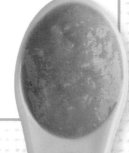

Papaya

Papaya, or pawpaw, is rich in protective vitamin C. Just half a small ripe pawpaw will make a simple purée for your baby. This is best prepared and served fresh.

  1–2 portions

ingredients

½ small ripe **papaya**

method

1 Remove and discard the black seeds from the fruit. Using a teaspoon, scoop out the pink flesh, discarding the skin.

2 Mash the flesh to make a purée.

3 Use immediately, then refrigerate any unused purée in an airtight container and use within 24 hours.

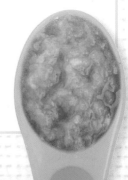

First *blends*

As your baby becomes used to single flavours, you can combine purées to make different dishes, either by mixing ones you have already made and frozen, or by trying out new recipes from this section. The more accustomed your baby becomes to eating from a spoon, the less runny the purée should be. Some of the recipes in this section include a tablespoon of vegetable oil. This ensures your baby gets calories and monounsaturated fats in addition to vitamins and some minerals from vegetables. After six months, you can continue to use your baby's usual milk in recipes, or use whole cow's milk, but don't give cow's milk as a drink until one year. As with the single tastes, where suitable for freezing, cool any remaining purée and freeze with the date and name of the food (see p58).

Carrot and pumpkin/ butternut squash

These autumn flavours are rich in vitamin A. Use frozen or prepared squash if you're not using the whole squash.

 8 mins 4 portions

ingredients

60g (2oz) or 1 small **carrot**, peeled and cut into cubes
100g (3½oz) peeled **butternut squash or pumpkin**, cut into cubes
1 tbsp **vegetable oil**

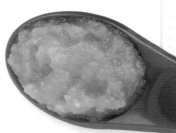

method

1 Steam the vegetables until they are tender, about 8 minutes. Cool slightly, then purée with the oil until smooth, adding your baby's usual milk, if needed.

Plum and apple

When plums are in season, this often forgotten fruit provides useful amounts of protective substances called polyphenols. Buy ripe plums that will be juicy and sweet.

 6–8 mins 5–6 portions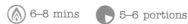

ingredients

1 medium **eating apple**, peeled, cored, and roughly chopped
2 medium **plums**, washed, stoned, and quartered

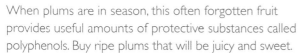

method

1 Place all the ingredients with 120ml (4fl oz) water in a small lidded saucepan and bring to the boil.

2 Stir, reduce the heat, and cover. Allow to simmer, stirring occasionally until the fruit is tender. Cool slightly, then purée.

Cauliflower and sweet potato

With vitamin C and folate, cauliflower pairs up well with vitamin A-rich sweet potato.

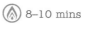 8–10 mins 4–5 portions

ingredients

150g (5½oz) or 1 small **sweet potato**, peeled and diced
70g (2½oz) or 2 **cauliflower** florets
1 tbsp **vegetable oil**
50ml (2fl oz) **milk**

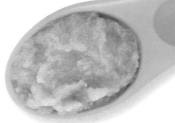

method

1 Steam the sweet potato and cauliflower until tender, around 8 minutes. Cool slightly, then blend with the oil and milk to make a thick purée.

Carrot, leek, and potato

These simple flavours are enhanced by gently frying the leek. The carrots are a cheap source of essential vitamin A.

 10–12 mins   5–6 portions   ❄

ingredients

8cm (3in) piece of **leek** – preferably the white part
1 tbsp **vegetable oil**
100g (3½oz) **carrots**, peeled and thinly sliced
120g (4oz) **potatoes**, peeled and quartered
milk, if needed

method

1 Slice the leek into small circles. Heat the oil in a small saucepan and gently fry the leek until soft.

2 Add the carrots and 100ml (3½fl oz) water, stir, and cover. Simmer gently until the carrots are soft, adding 1–2 tablespoons more water if required.

3 Meanwhile, steam the potatoes until tender. Press them through a ricer into a clean bowl, or use a potato masher.

4 Purée the carrot and leek and stir into the mashed potato, adding a little milk if you need to adjust the texture.

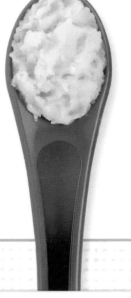

Courgette, spinach, and tomato

As weaning progresses and there's more food to prepare, you won't want to spend more time than is necessary in the kitchen. Skinning and seeding tomatoes can be avoided by using a bottle or carton of long-life unsalted sieved passata. This is heat-treated in its preparation so doesn't require further cooking, making it easy to add while puréeing. Tomatoes provide valuable vitamin C, which helps the body to absorb iron.

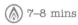 7–8 mins   5–6 portions   ❄

ingredients

1 tbsp **vegetable oil**
100g (3½oz) **courgettes**, washed and cut into cubes
100g (3½oz) **spinach leaves**, rinsed
50–75ml (1¾–2½fl oz) **passata**
pinch of **ground nutmeg** (optional)

method

1 Heat the oil in a saucepan and cook the courgettes without browning until just soft.

2 Add the spinach leaves, stir, and cover. Continue to cook over a low heat for 3–4 minutes until the spinach has wilted, then remove from the heat.

3 Purée the courgette and spinach mixture and then stir in as much passata as you need for an appropriate texture. Stir in the nutmeg if using.

* Tip: *You can stir in a little baby rice to adjust the texture if the purée is too runny.*

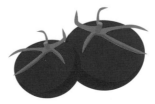

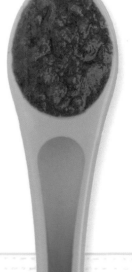

Broccoli, pea, and potato

Most babies enjoy potato and it makes the texture transition from runny purées to thicker foods easy. As potato doesn't purée well, use a potato ricer, or masher, mixing in milk or oil before stirring in other vegetables.

 8–10 mins   5–6 portions

ingredients

100g (3½oz) **potatoes**, peeled and quartered
100g (3½oz) **broccoli** florets, washed
50g (1¾oz) frozen **peas**
1 tbsp **vegetable oil**
milk, if needed

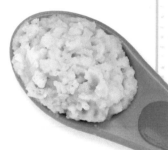

method

1 Steam or boil the potatoes until tender.

2 Meanwhile, steam the broccoli and peas together until tender.

3 In a clean bowl, press the potatoes through a ricer, or use a potato masher if you prefer, and stir in the oil.

4 Blend the peas and broccoli to make a purée, adding milk if necessary, and stir into the mashed potato.

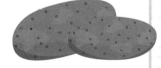

Parsnip and sweet potato

A sweet root vegetable combination, sweet potato is a fabulous source of vitamin A as well as providing essential vitamins E and C. Choose smaller parsnips as large ones tend to be a bit woody in the centre.

 10–12 mins   6–8 portions

ingredients

100g (3½oz) **parsnips**, peeled and cut into chunks
200g (7oz) **sweet potatoes**, peeled and cut into chunks
50–75ml (1¾–2½fl oz) **milk**

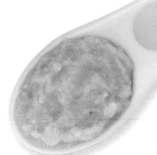

method

1 Steam the parsnips and sweet potatoes together until they are both tender.

2 Cool slightly, then purée with the milk to create a smooth consistency.

* Tip: *This purée can be added to mashed potato, or used to add to stews or soups, where it will help thicken the dish as well as provide essential nutrients.*

Sweetcorn, squash, and tomato

This makes a lovely transition to a more textured purée, and is a good source of vitamins A, C, and B3 (niacin).

 12 mins   3–4 portions

ingredients

75g (2½oz) **butternut squash**, peeled and diced
75g (2½oz) frozen **sweetcorn**
60ml (2fl oz) or 4 tbsp **passata**
1 tbsp **vegetable oil**

method

1 Steam the squash for 10 minutes, then add the sweetcorn and cook until tender.

2 Cool slightly, then blend with the passata and oil to make a thick purée.

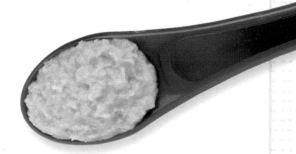

Apricot and pear

This sweet fruity mix is a healthy treat for your baby, packed with vitamins C and E.

 10–15 mins   10 portions   ❄

ingredients

100g (3½ oz)
   ready-to-eat **apricots**
2 medium ripe **pears**,
   peeled, cored and
   diced
250ml 8fl oz) **water**

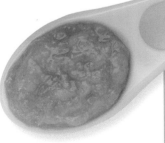

method

1 Place the dried apricots in a small saucepan and pour over the water. Cover and bring to the boil, then simmer until the apricots are soft. Cool slightly.

2 Meanwhile, steam the pears for 5–6 minutes.

3 Combine the ingredients, together with the cooking liquid, then purée.

Avocado and banana

This classic combination is a favourite with babies. Rich in vitamin E and healthy monounsaturated fat, avocado, like banana, is easily portable for a meal on the move.

🚫 1 portion

ingredients

¼ ripe **avocado**, sliced
¼ ripe **banana**, sliced

method

1 Mash the avocado and banana with a fork until you have a smooth purée.

2 Use immediately.

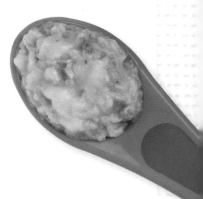

Broccoli, leek, and potato

As you build up your baby's repertoire of vegetables, you can try adding leeks or spring onions, gently fried for flavour, as in this recipe.

 8–10 mins   6–7 portions   ❄

ingredients

1 tbsp **vegetable oil**
50g (1¾oz) **leeks**,
   washed and thinly sliced
150g (5½oz) **potatoes**,
   peeled and quartered

150g (5½oz) **broccoli**
   florets, washed
milk, if needed

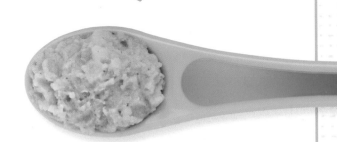

method

1 Heat the oil in a small saucepan and gently cook the leeks, for about 5 minutes, stirring often until softened, but not browned. Remove from the heat.

2 Meanwhile, steam or boil the potatoes until tender, about 5 minutes. Steam the broccoli until tender, then purée with the leeks, adding milk if needed.

3 In a clean bowl, press the potatoes through a ricer, or use a potato masher, and mix with the leek and broccoli mixture.

Breakfasts

You can introduce variety into your baby's breakfasts by combining fruit purées with cereals or yogurts. Shop-bought baby porridge or cereal is made from oats or a mixture of other gluten-free cereals. These baby cereals contain milk powder from follow-on milk and are usually fortified with vitamins and sometimes minerals. Make sure you follow the instructions on the packet and don't add milk unless you are instructed to do so. For early weaning, you can make your own baby porridge with grains you have at home if you prefer: whizz rolled oat flakes or porridge oats into a fine flour in your processor or blender. As your baby gets used to solids, you can try giving him unblended flakes.

Yogurt with cinnamon and pear

Yogurt is a good source of calcium and magnesium for bones and teeth. Stirring in a pinch of cinnamon makes this fruit and yogurt combo a little different for your baby.

  1 portion

ingredients

2 tbsp full-fat **plain yogurt**
2 tsp **pear purée** (see p59)
pinch of **ground cinnamon**

method

1 Mix together the yogurt, pear, and cinnamon and serve immediately.

Apple and yogurt breakfast

Full-fat plain yogurt can be mixed with a variety of simple purées. Apple is added here, but you can also try mango, banana or blueberry, or whichever purée you fancy, to make a nutritious start to the day.

1 portion

ingredients

2 tbsp full-fat **plain yogurt**
2 tsp **apple purée** (see p59)

method

1 Mix together the yogurt and apple, or other fruit, and serve immediately.

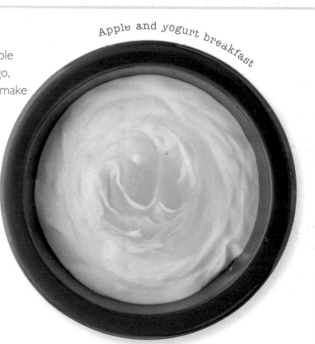

Apple and yogurt breakfast

Apricot porridge

Porridge made with flaked oats may be too lumpy for your baby to start with, but you can easily make it into a finer grain by whizzing in the processor.

 2–3 mins   1 portion

ingredients

15g (½oz) or 1 tbsp **oat flour,** or **flakes** for an older baby

75ml (2½fl oz) **baby's usual milk**

1 tbsp **apricot purée** (see p60)

method

1 Place the oats and milk in a small saucepan and heat, stirring constantly.

2 When the mixture thickens, remove from the heat and cool to body temperature.

3 Stir in the apricot purée and serve immediately.

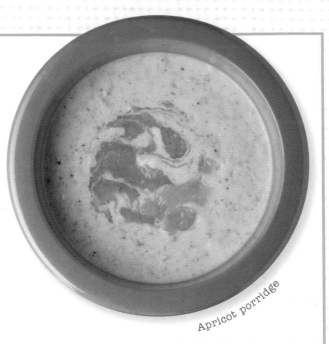

Apricot porridge

Banana oat porridge

Comforting nutritious porridge with a hint of banana is quick and easy to make and a lovely way for your baby to start the day.

 2–3 mins   1 portion

ingredients

15g (½oz) or 1 tbsp **oat flour,** or **flakes** for an older baby

75ml (2½fl oz) **baby's usual milk**

few slices of **banana**

method

1 Place the oats and milk in a small saucepan and heat, stirring constantly.

2 When the mixture thickens, remove from the heat and cool to body temperature.

3 Meanwhile, mash the banana with a fork until smooth and stir into the porridge.

* Microwave version: *Mix the oats and milk in a microwaveable bowl and cook on a high heat for 30 seconds (800W oven). Stir and cook for another 10 seconds. (The timing will vary according to the power of your oven.) Once thickened, remove from the oven, stir, and allow to cool before adding the banana.*

Millet and banana porridge

Millet is a gluten-free grain that makes a simple first breakfast, providing iron and vitamin B3. Millet flakes or flour are perfect for this simple porridge.

 2–3 mins   1 portion

ingredients

15g (½oz) or 1 tbsp **millet flour** or **flakes**

75ml (2½fl oz) **baby's usual milk**

few slices of **banana**

method

1 Place the millet and milk in a small saucepan and heat, stirring constantly.

2 When the mixture thickens, remove from the heat and cool to body temperature.

3 Meanwhile, mash the banana with a fork until smooth and stir into the porridge.

* Tip: *For a bigger appetite, simply double the ingredients.*

Hard-boiled egg

Storing eggs in the fridge will keep them fresh. Make sure eggs are well cooked in the early stages of weaning.

 10 mins   1 portion

ingredients

1 fresh **egg**

method

1 Fill a small saucepan with enough water to cover an egg. Bring to the boil.

2 Gently lower the egg into the saucepan, being careful not to knock its shell. Boil for around 10 minutes.

3 Leave to cool, then remove the shell and slice the egg into quarters for your baby.

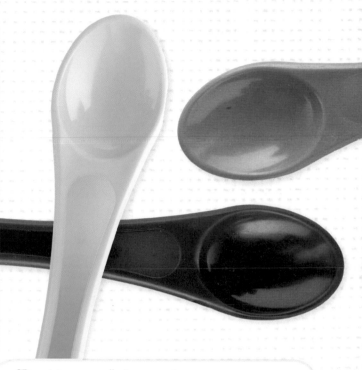

Buttered toast

Once your baby is able to hold foods, he can enjoy some toast fingers. He may find white or wholemeal bread easier to eat at first than bread with cracked grains or seeds. Use a monounsaturated spread such as olive, or unsalted butter if you prefer, or try full-fat cream cheese. Your baby may like to dip his toast into a fruit purée.

 2 mins   1 portion

ingredients

½ slice **white** or **wholemeal bread**

olive spread or **unsalted butter**

method

1 Toast the bread, then cut it into 2–3 sections to make toast fingers.

2 Spread with the chosen topping.

Buttered toast

Fromage frais and fruit purée

Buy unsweetened plain fromage frais and make your own fruity version by adding one of the fruit purées you've made already. Your baby needs full-fat fromage frais to provide essential calories.

  1 portion

ingredients

2 tbsp **full-fat fromage frais**
2 tsp **fruit purée** (see pp59–62)

method

1 Mix together the fromage frais and purée and serve immediately.

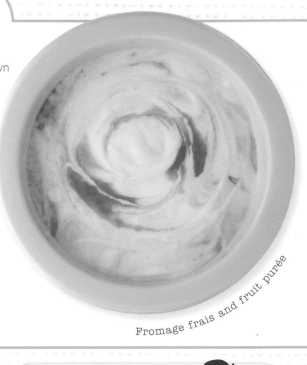

Fromage frais and fruit purée

Wheat biscuit with milk

Wheat biscuits are a popular first breakfast as they soak up milk easily and quickly become soft, making them simple for your baby to eat. Use either specially formulated baby wheat biscuits, or standard ones.

  1 portion

ingredients

½ **wheat biscuit**
60ml (2fl oz) or 4 tbsp of your **baby's usual**

milk, or whole milk (after six months), cold or warmed

method

1 Crumble the wheat biscuit into a bowl and pour over the milk.

2 Allow to soften for a couple of minutes, and stir. Serve immediately.

Orchard fruits breakfast

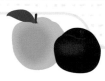

Vary your baby's breakfasts by adding different fruit purées to wheat biscuits.

  1 portion

ingredients

½ **wheat biscuit**
60ml (2fl oz) or 4 tbsp of your **baby's usual milk** or **whole milk**

(after six months), cold or warmed
1 tbsp **plum and apple purée** (see p63)

method

1 Crumble the wheat biscuit into a bowl and pour over the milk.

2 Allow to soften for a couple of minutes, then stir in the plum and apple purée. Serve immediately.

★ Tip: *If you have frozen portions of fruit purée, pop one in a bowl and defrost in the microwave before you start. Or if you are very organized, defrost in the fridge the night before.*

First *meals*

When your baby has become used to eating food from a spoon and accepts a range of different single and blended flavours, it's important to introduce more protein-rich foods such as meat, poultry, fish, beans, and cheese into his diet. Meat, fish, poultry, and beans all contain iron, essential for his growth and development (pp14–17). If you've waited until six months to start weaning, make sure you introduce these iron-rich purées within a couple of weeks. See page 27 for advice on freezing additional portions.

Cauliflower, cheese, and potato

A good source of calcium and vitamin C, sauce-rich cauliflower cheese is a family favourite.

 5 mins   10–15 mins

5–6 portions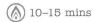

ingredients

100g (3½oz) **potatoes**, peeled and cut into chunks
200g (7oz) **cauliflower** florets, washed

75ml (2½fl oz) **milk**
40g (1½oz) **Cheddar cheese**, grated

method

1 Steam the potatoes and cauliflower together until tender.

2 Using tongs, remove the cauliflower and purée with the milk in a blender until smooth.

3 Press the potatoes through a ricer into a clean bowl, or use a potato masher, and stir in the cheese.

4 Mix together the potato and cauliflower mixtures. Cool slightly before serving.

Potato, spinach, and ricotta

Ricotta is a mild soft cheese, which adds protein and calcium to this yummy mixture. You can add milk or water to adjust the texture if this is too firm.

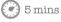 5 mins    5–6 portions   10–15 mins

ingredients

200g (7oz) **potatoes**
1 tbsp **vegetable oil**
2 **spring onions**, trimmed, washed, and cut into small pieces
100g (3½oz) **spinach leaves**, washed and drained
50g (1¾oz) **ricotta cheese**
pinch of grated **nutmeg** (optional)

method

1 Peel the potatoes, cut into chunks, and steam until soft, about 5 minutes.

2 Meanwhile, heat the oil in a medium saucepan and gently cook the spring onions until soft, without browning them.

3 Add the spinach, cover, and cook for 3–4 minutes until the spinach has wilted.

4 Press the cooked potato through a ricer or mash until soft, and stir in the ricotta cheese.

5 Purée the spinach and onion mixture and stir into the cheesy potato along with a pinch of grated nutmeg if using. Cool slightly before serving.

* Variation: *If you prefer, you can use 20g (¾oz) leeks instead of spring onions.*

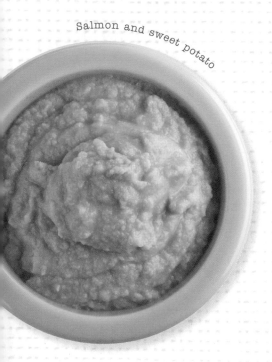

Salmon and sweet potato

Salmon and sweet potato

Salmon is a popular oily fish, providing essential omega 3 fatty acids for your baby's eye and brain development. Mixed with sweet potato and carrots, this colourful meal is likely to become a firm favourite.

 5 mins 15–17 mins 6–8 portions ❄

ingredients

200g (7oz) **sweet potatoes**, peeled and cut into 1cm (½in) cubes
100g (3½oz) or 1 large **carrot**, peeled and cut into 1cm (½in) cubes

75g (2½oz) skinless **salmon fillet**
120ml (4fl oz) cooled and boiled **water** or **milk**

method

1 Place the sweet potato and carrot pieces in a steamer over a pan of boiling water and cook for 5 minutes.

2 Meanwhile, run your finger over the fish to check for any bones, removing any you find. Loosely wrap the fish in a piece of foil and place it on top of the vegetables. Continue steaming for 10–12 minutes.

3 Remove the parcel of fish and check if it is cooked by inserting a knife to separate the flakes. The fish should look opaque and be the same colour throughout. If it isn't, return to the pan and steam for a few minutes more.

4 Check if the vegetables are tender, and remove from the pan to cool slightly.

5 Mix the salmon, sweet potato, and carrots in a blender with the water or milk to make a smooth purée.

* Variation: *Use a trout fillet instead of salmon.*

Cod, pea, and potato

You can substitute the cod here for other responsibly sourced fish such as haddock, whiting, coley or pollock. These white fish are simple to cook and easy for your baby to digest. Using peas adds sweetness and is a good step on the way to your baby enjoying fish pie with the rest of the family.

 5 mins 12–15 mins 7–10 portions ❄

ingredients

200g (7oz) **potatoes**, peeled and cut into 1–2 cm (½–¾in) cubes
100g (3½oz) skinless **cod fillet** ¼ tsp finely chopped **mint** (optional)
150g (5½oz) frozen **petit pois**
75ml (2½fl oz) **milk**, plus more if needed
2 tsp **monounsaturate-rich spread** (such as olive)

method

1 Place the potatoes in a steamer and cook for 5 minutes, or until tender.

2 Meanwhile, run your finger over the fish to check for any bones, removing any you find. Loosely wrap the fish in a piece of foil and sprinkle over the mint, if using.

3 Place the peas in a separate steamer with the fish parcel over it, and steam for 6–7 minutes.

4 Remove the fish parcel and the peas, and check the fish is cooked by inserting a knife to separate the flakes. The fish should look opaque and be the same colour throughout. If it isn't, steam it again until it is cooked through.

5 Mash the potatoes with 40ml (1½fl oz) of the milk, and the spread. Purée the peas and fish together with the remaining milk, adding more if required, and mix together with the potatoes.

Butterbean, parsnip, and sweet potato

A lovely introduction to pulses, butterbeans taste fairly bland and combine nicely with the sweet potato and parsnips.

 5 mins   10–12 mins  5–6 portions ❄

ingredients

50g (1¾oz) **parsnips**, peeled and diced
100g (3½oz) **sweet potatoes**, peeled and diced
200g (7oz) can **butterbeans** in water,

drained and rinsed
a few sprigs of **parsley**, rinsed
1 tbsp **vegetable oil**
65ml (2fl oz) cooled boiled **water** or **milk**

method

1 Place the parsnips and sweet potatoes in a steamer and cook for 5 minutes, or until almost tender.

2 Add the butterbeans and parsley and steam for another 3–4 minutes to heat through.

3 Purée with the oil and milk or water until smooth.

Lentil, tomato, and coriander dhal

This simple dhal provides protein as well as iron and vitamin C for your baby. Serve it alone or thicken with baby rice or mashed potato. As weaning progresses to include more lumpy food, you can mash rather than purée this dish.

 5 mins   20–25 mins

 4 portions ❄

ingredients

1 tbsp **vegetable oil**
25g (scant 1oz) **onions**, finely chopped
50g (1¾oz) **split red lentils**

200g (7oz) chopped canned **tomatoes**
pinch of **ground coriander**
1 tsp chopped fresh **coriander** (optional)

method

1 Heat the oil in a non-stick saucepan and fry the onion for 3–4 minutes until softened. Stir in the lentils, tomatoes, and ground coriander.

2 Add 200ml (7fl oz) of water and bring the mixture to the boil. Reduce the heat, cover, and simmer for 15–20 minutes until the lentils are soft.

3 Stir in the fresh coriander and cook for another 1–2 minutes. Remove from the heat and cool slightly before puréeing.

✱ **Tip:** If you are using fresh herbs, make sure that they are washed and patted dry on kitchen paper. Add green herbs in the last few minutes of cooking so that the heat destroys any food-poisoning bacteria.

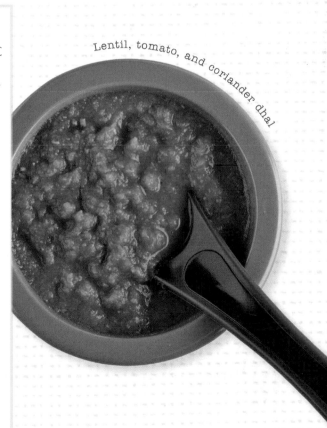
Lentil, tomato, and coriander dhal

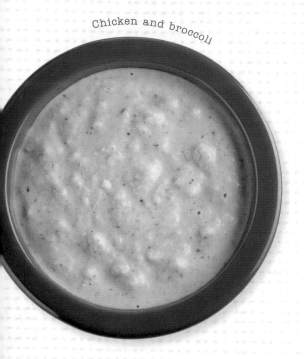

Chicken and broccoli

Chicken and broccoli

Your baby will already be familiar with broccoli; combining this with chicken provides a protein-rich meal. You can serve this dish on its own or thicken it with a little baby rice to make a more complete meal.

 5–6 mins 8–10 mins

 6–8 portions ❄

ingredients

1 tbsp **vegetable oil**
100g (3½oz) **chicken mince**

200g (7oz) **broccoli** florets
90ml (3fl oz) cooled and boiled **water** or **milk**

method

1 Heat the oil in a small saucepan and gently fry the mince for 2 minutes before stirring in 75ml (2½fl oz) water.

2 Cover and simmer for 5 minutes, or until the mince is cooked through.

3 Steam the broccoli florets until tender. Purée the mince with any cooking liquid, and add the broccoli. Blend with the remaining water or milk until smooth.

* Tip: *If you are adding baby rice, mix in 1 heaped teaspoon of baby rice for each tablespoon of the purée.*

Beef, carrot, and potato

Beef is a good source of iron and zinc so it is an important protein-rich food to introduce to your baby at around six months of age. Choose lean minced beef as this is lower in saturated fats, and fry it in healthy monounsaturated vegetable (rapeseed) oil.

 5–10 mins 18–20 mins 8–10 portions ❄

ingredients

1 tbsp **vegetable oil**
100g (3½oz) lean **beef mince**
200g (7oz) **carrots**, peeled, quartered, and sliced
200g (7oz) **potatoes**, peeled and diced
milk to blend, if needed

method

1 Heat the oil in a saucepan and gently fry the mince for 2–3 minutes until lightly browned.

2 Add the carrots to the mince along with 200ml (7fl oz) water, and bring to the boil. Stir, cover, and reduce the heat. Allow to simmer for 15 minutes, or until the carrots are soft.

3 Meanwhile, steam or boil the potatoes. Purée the carrots, beef, and cooking water until smooth.

4 Press the cooked potatoes through a ricer or mouli, or mash finely using a little milk if needed. Mix the potatoes with the beef and the carrots.

* Tip: *As the potato is cooked alone, you can freeze the beef and carrot mixture separately if you prefer. By pulsing the blender or processor, you can achieve a rougher purée, which is useful for stage 2 weaning.*

* Variations: *Use lamb instead of beef mince. Add ¼ teaspoon dried mixed herbs at stage 3.*

Lamb and apricots

Lamb, like beef, provides easily absorbed iron and zinc. The addition of tomatoes here ensures there is vitamin C to help your baby absorb the iron. You can use this purée alongside mashed potato, with rice, or in the later stages of weaning with couscous.

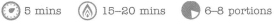

5 mins   15–20 mins   6–8 portions

ingredients

100g (3½oz) **lamb mince**
50g (1¾oz) ready-to-eat
   apricots, halved if large
200g (7oz) **passata**
pinch of **ground cinnamon**

method

1 Place the mince in a small non-stick saucepan and gently brown in its own fat over a low heat for 2–3 minutes, stirring constantly to break up the mince.

2 Add the apricots, passata, and 100ml (3½fl oz) water. Sprinkle in the cinnamon, stir, and cover.

3 Simmer gently for 10–15 minutes, stirring occasionally, until the mince is cooked through and the apricots are tender. Cool the mixture slightly, then purée.

4 Serve with baby rice, potato, or sweet potato.

✱ Tip: You can use a 200g (7oz) can of chopped tomatoes in juice instead of passata.

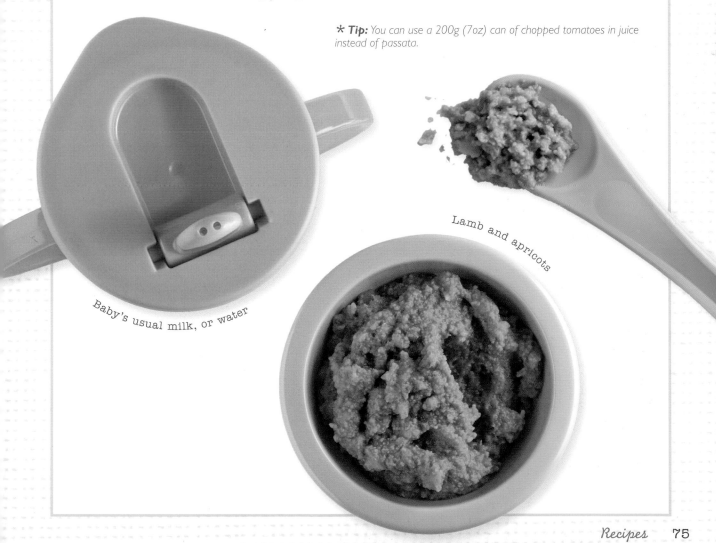

Baby's usual milk, or water

Lamb and apricots

Introducing *Stage 2*

In the second stage of weaning, around seven to nine months, your baby's ability to grasp objects improves, and she may hold a spoon, pick up soft finger foods, and gets used to holding a spouted cup. She eats two to three meals a day, which play an increasingly important role nutritionally. As her muscles strengthen, she sits more upright in a high chair, giving her a good view of what's going on at mealtimes.

Progressing through the second stage

The texture of your baby's meals changes during this stage from puréed food to mashed food (if you haven't done this already), food with soft lumps, and minced foods. She will also be eating a range of finger foods.

Her ability to chew improves during this stage, whether or not she has any teeth, so it's vital that she is introduced to lumps in food as well as dissolving or soft finger foods so she can practise chewing. Start by introducing soft lumps in familiar foods, such as well-cooked potato and vegetables. Tiny pasta shapes are also ideal lumpy foods that will encourage her to chew. She can progress onto larger lumps and slightly harder textures, including finger foods, over the weeks. Don't delay this phase for fear that she might choke: it's important for her to manage soft lumps by the time she is nine months old, otherwise she may become resistant to trying new textures if left too long.

Continuity and perseverance are important during this stage. Carry on offering savoury foods and vegetables in preference to desserts or fruit, so that your baby doesn't reject savoury in favour of sweet.

What your baby eats now

- Milk, whether breast or formula, is still vital to your baby. In this stage, as your baby starts to eat larger amounts of foods, the amount of milk she wants may go down a little, although she shouldn't have less than around 500ml (two to four breastfeeds) a day. If you decide to start weaning your baby from breastfeeding now, make sure you choose a suitable formula milk as an alternative (see p47).

- By this second stage of weaning, your baby should be eating meals that contain meat, fish or poultry once a day. These provide essential protein, B vitamins, iron, zinc, and omega 3 fatty acids, which milk alone doesn't supply adequately for your growing baby. The menu plans will help you to introduce nutrient-rich foods such as lamb, chicken, beef, cod, salmon, and tofu.

- Vegetarian babies need a mixture of pulses, tofu, nut and seed butters, cheese, and eggs to provide different vegetarian sources of protein. You could also talk to a health visitor about giving an omega 3 supplement.

- Although milk is still vital, you may be giving other drinks, too; there's advice on pages 46–7 on which drinks are suitable for your baby.

 Timing meals and milk feeds

When your baby's daily meal quota goes up, you may need to alter the timing of her milk feeds so she has an appetite for food. Mornings are tricky as your baby wakes up hungry and may be used to a large milk feed. If this is her routine, you could give her a milk feed first thing, then delay her breakfast until you are up and ready for the day. If she has a large feed late morning, try splitting this so she has some before lunch and the rest after lunch (perhaps giving two smaller bottles or offering just one breast at a time). As you progress, you will probably find you develop a pattern of regular meals that fit around sleep and activities.

STAGE 2 – at a glance

TEXTURE

During the second stage of weaning, the texture of your baby's food should progress from **mashed food** to **chopped textures** and **soft** or **dissolving** finger foods.

INTRODUCE

You can now introduce: cow's milk in cooking · more pasta products · soft berries · soya and tofu products · nuts.*
*Note: if you have a family history of allergies, consult your GP before giving your baby nuts.

AVOID

Don't give processed meats, such as sausages and ham, honey, liver, and whole nuts (see p19).

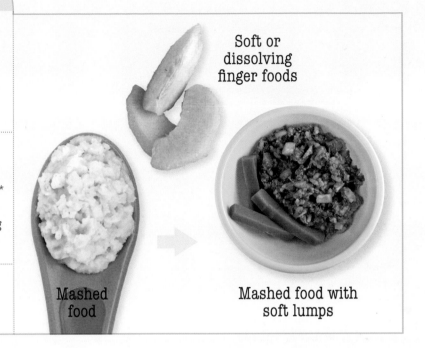

Mashed food

Soft or dissolving finger foods

Mashed food with soft lumps

Portion sizes

The table below is a guide to the usual portion sizes for babies during stage 2, although individual babies will differ on the amount they need to eat. It assumes that foods from the main food groups are mixed together.

FOODS	TYPICAL MEAL	TYPICAL AMOUNT FOR 7–9 MONTH OLD
Cereal mixed with milk	Breakfast	5 teaspoons to 5 tablespoons per meal
Fruit purée with dairy	Dessert or breakfast	5 teaspoons
Savoury dish including vegetables, protein source (meat, poultry, fish, eggs or pulses) and pasta, potatoes or rice	Lunch or dinner	5–10 teaspoons per meal
Dairy – milk dessert	Dessert – lunch or dinner	5–10 teaspoons
Milk – formula or breastfeed	Throughout day	500–600ml (17fl oz–1 pint) formula milk or
Finger foods	With meals	Half slice bread or 1 rice cake, 2 pieces pasta, 2–3 pieces softened fruit or vegetables
High-fat and high-sugar foods	Not suitable	Not suitable

Hands *on*

Finger foods come into their own from stage 2 onwards as your baby's hand–eye coordination improves. Eating whole foods also helps her learn to chew efficiently, which in turn is an important part of speech development as she learns to coordinate the muscles needed for talking. Her control over her fingers and thumb improves now, so a chair with an attached tray is helpful as you can place finger foods straight on the tray for her to attempt to grasp.

Introducing finger foods

Soft fruits are perfect first finger foods, cut into pieces that are big enough for your baby to pick up and easy to eat. You may have already introduced these towards the end of stage 1, so can build up your baby's repertoire now. Make sure you remove any pips or stones from fruits. You can also start to serve cooked vegetable finger foods alongside your baby's meals. Cut vegetables into batons, slices, or florets, and steam or oven bake them until soft. Over time, and as your baby's chewing skills develop, some of these can be introduced raw.

There are plenty of commercial baby snack foods that make great finger foods and can come in handy when you are out and about. However, try to resist the temptation to comfort or distract your baby at home with baby breadsticks and bite-and-dissolve snacks as these may spoil her appetite for meals.

"I want to do it!"

Enjoying finger foods is an important part of learning to self-feed, giving your baby the chance to develop independent eating habits. If your baby was resistant to being spoon-fed, being able to feed herself finger foods allows her more control and can make mealtimes easier for you both. If you have followed the baby-led weaning route, you will have introduced finger foods from an earlier age, allowing your baby to select from a range of foods offered on her high-chair tray.

Take care

- Stay with your baby at all times when she is eating new textures and finger foods in case she chokes (see p39 on how to prepare foods to prevent choking).

- Be careful with dried fruit, as this can stick to teeth, increasing the risk of decay. Raisins are best left for mealtimes, unless you clean your baby's teeth afterwards. You can soak dried fruit in a little water first to soften it.

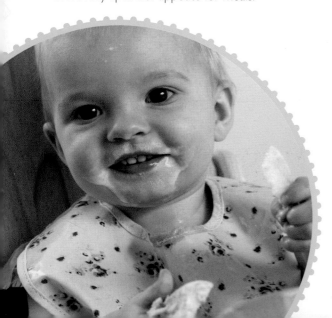

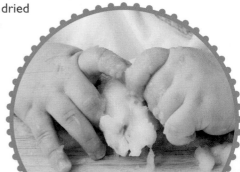

10 easy-to-prepare finger foods

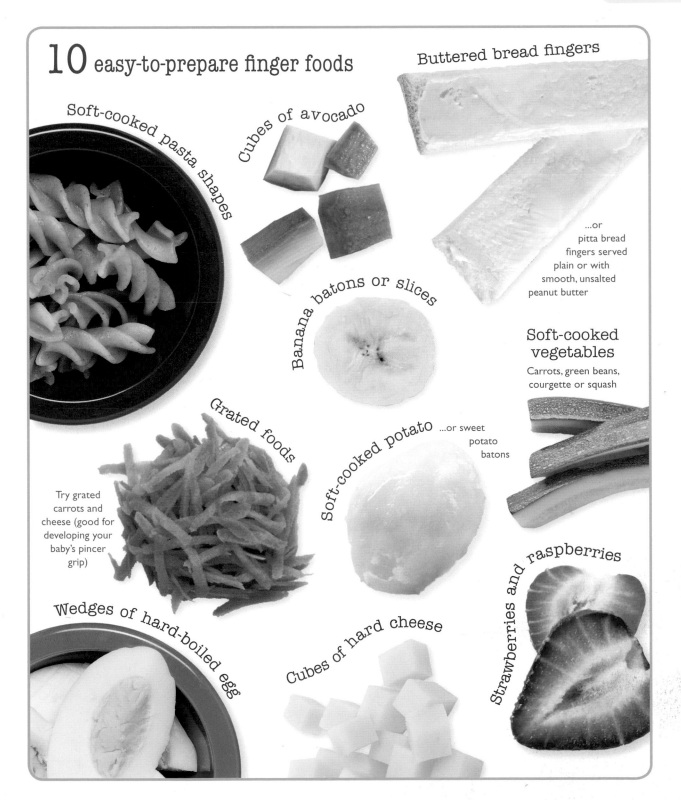

Soft-cooked pasta shapes

Cubes of avocado

Buttered bread fingers

...or pitta bread fingers served plain or with smooth, unsalted peanut butter

Banana batons or slices

Soft-cooked vegetables

Carrots, green beans, courgette or squash

Grated foods

Soft-cooked potato

...or sweet potato batons

Try grated carrots and cheese (good for developing your baby's pincer grip)

Wedges of hard-boiled egg

Cubes of hard cheese

Strawberries and raspberries

Eating *out*

As you and your baby develop a routine, you will be taking her out and about to meet friends and family, go shopping, or take trips to the park, which can mean being out during mealtimes. There are plenty of ideas for healthy, portable meals.

Making the planner work away from home

The menu planner contains plenty of recipes that can be eaten cold. By swapping days around to suit your schedule, it's easy to make the planner work for you and your baby when you're away from home. Some portable foods include:

- Apricot and pear purée (p66)
- Avocado purée (p61)
- Banana purée (p59)
- Avocado and banana purée (p66)
- Home-made hummus (p111) with cooled steamed vegetables (pp118–19)
- Cottage cheese dip (p107) with baby breadsticks or pitta bread fingers
- Baby falafel (p110) with tzatziki

- Banana custard (p133)
- Creamy apricot dessert (p129)
- Yogurt with stewed fruit (p129)

As your baby grows and starts to eat more complete meals, you can try:

- Baby pizzas (pp178–9)
- Fruity couscous (p102) and cottage cheese or cheese cubes
- Hard-boiled egg wedges (p69), cherry tomatoes, and bread and butter
- Baby blueberry pancakes (p169) spread with soft cheese
- Baby egg and cress sandwich (p175) with red pepper fingers
- Pasta – filled or plain
- Apply plums (p129)
- Rice pudding (p135) with mandarins

Staying safe

When you're eating away from home, don't relax on safety and hygiene:

- Clean yours and your baby's hands before eating.
- When transporting home-made food, pack a bowl and several spoons so you can use one spoon for placing food in the bowl and the other spoon for feeding your baby. This ensures your baby's saliva doesn't contaminate food that hasn't been decanted.
- If you are using a jar of food, throw away any that remains uneaten that you can't refrigerate – it isn't safe to use commercial food that has been opened and not eaten unless it is refrigerated straight away.
- Don't give your baby a pouch of food to suck while she's sitting in her buggy. Your baby doesn't use her tongue to control food while sucking, so she is more likely to choke on a lump while sucking a pouch. Wait until you've stopped for lunch, then decant the pouch into a bowl.
- Never give your baby food to eat while you're driving unless there's an adult sitting next to her.

Using shop-bought foods

It's undoubtedly convenient to pack an unopened jar or pouch of baby food for days out, and shop-bought baby foods can add variety to your baby's diet. If an item is from the supermarket shelf rather than a fresh refrigerated food, it doesn't need special storage. It can be served at room temperature or, if you are in a restaurant or someone's home, you can ask for it to be heated.

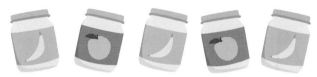

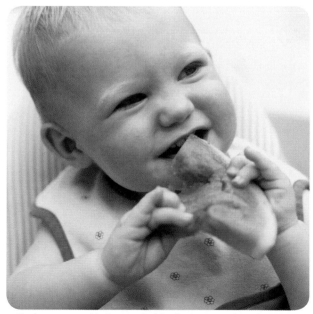

Easily transportable fruit is ideal for feeding away from home.

Eating in restaurants

Some restaurants are more baby-friendly than others, so it's worth finding out in advance what, if any, provision they make for little visitors. Check the following:

- Do they provide high chairs?

- Does the restaurant provide toys or crayons to keep older babies and children amused? If not, take some quiet toys along to keep her occupied; choose ones that will sit easily on the high-chair tray.

- Are there items on the menu that may be suitable for your baby, such as foods that you could mash with a fork or cut finely, or that she can pick up and eat herself. Avoid any food with added salt.

- If the restaurant doesn't have suitable foods on the menu, will they heat commercially bought baby food? (They are unlikely to heat home-made food because of the risk your food could pose.) Do they provide their own jars of baby food that they will heat up?

- Do they mind if you bring along some cold foods for your baby to eat at the table?

- Coffee shops rarely provide suitable foods for babies, so if you're planning to stop off at one on a trip out, take your own food or choose a simple sandwich.

day-by-day meal planner
Week 1

Offer your baby a drink with her meals – either her usual milk or water in a lidded cup. If you wish to give juice, give unsweetened fruit juice diluted one part juice to 10 parts water.

Monday

Breakfast
Apricot porridge p68

Lunch
Italian tomato and tuna mash p120

Dinner
Beef and onion casserole p116 with mashed potato
Banana custard p133

Tuesday

Breakfast
Wheat biscuit p70 with apple purée p59/milk

Lunch
Cod, pea, and potato p72

Dinner
Chicken and broccoli p74 with rice
Papaya fingers p131

Wednesday

Breakfast
Millet and banana porridge p68

Lunch
Hard-boiled egg with buttered toast p69

Dinner
Cheesy mash with fish and peas p117
Creamy apricot dessert p129

Thursday

Breakfast
Apricot and pear purée p66 with buttered toast p69

Lunch
Tofu and avocado dip p108

Dinner
Italian tomato and tuna mash p120
Yogurt with fruit purée p96

Friday

Breakfast
Mango purée and yogurt p67

Lunch
Cheesy mash with fish and peas p117

Dinner
Yummy veggie sauce with pasta p122
Chocolate rice pudding p135

Saturday

Breakfast
Apple and raspberries p97 with yogurt

Lunch
Home-made hummus p111 with steamed vegetables pp118–19

Dinner
Lamb and apricots p75 with rice and cooked spinach
Stewed apple and cranberries p129

Sunday

Breakfast
Banana oat porridge p68

Lunch
Beef and onion casserole p116 with mashed potato

Dinner
Creamy salmon and pasta p121
Fruit fool p133

Other ideas this week Raspberry porridge p99 • Carrot and lentil soup p103 • Sweet potato, barley, and leek soup p102 • Cauliflower cheese p125 with bread and butter • Fruity chicken p112 with mashed potato • Mango lollies p132 • Halved grapes and pear slices p130

day-by-day meal planner
Week 2

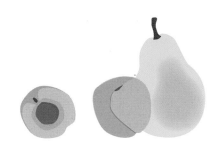

Monday
Breakfast
Fromage frais and sliced banana

Lunch
Home-made hummus p111 with steamed vegetables pp118–19 and pitta

Dinner
Lamb and apricots p75 with rice and broccoli
Fruit fool p133

Tuesday
Breakfast
Banana oat porridge p68

Lunch
Hard-boiled egg with buttered toast p69

Dinner
Fruity chicken p112 with mashed sweet potato
Yogurt with fruit purée p96

Wednesday
Breakfast
Wheat biscuit p70 with apple purée p59/milk

Lunch
Sweet potato, barley, and leek soup p102

Dinner
Cod, pea, and potato p72
Ground rice pudding p134

Thursday
Breakfast
Yogurt and pear slices p130

Lunch
Chicken and broccoli p74 with rice

Dinner
Creamy salmon and pasta p121
Fruit fool p133

Friday
Breakfast
Millet porridge p68 with apple purée p59

Lunch
Cottage cheese dip p107 with steamed vegetables pp118–19

Dinner
Coconut lentil dhal p128 with rice
Berries with chocolate dipping sauce p135

Saturday
Breakfast
Spicy plum and banana p96

Lunch
Sweet potatoes with sardines and peas p117

Dinner
Greek baked fish p120 with mashed potato
Soft pear slices p130

Sunday
Breakfast
Date Porridge p98

Lunch
Avocado dip p105 with bread

Dinner
Normandy pork p113 with mashed potato
Banana custard p133

Other ideas this week
French toast p98 and fruit purée pp59–62 • Oat porridge p98 • Yummy veggie sauce with pasta p122 • Butternut squash risotto p122 • Beef ragu p115 with pasta shapes and broccoli florets • Garden vegetable risotto p127 • Apply plums p129

day-by-day meal planner
Week 3

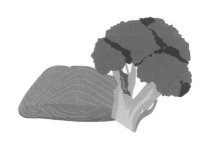

Monday

Breakfast
Hard-boiled egg with buttered toast p69

Lunch
Flaked fish p106 with avocado dip p105

Dinner
Tofu with spinach and rice p127
Fruits of the forest iced yogurt p133

Tuesday

Breakfast
Apricot and pear purée p66 with fromage frais

Lunch
Italian tomato and tuna mash p120

Dinner
Baby's first lamb tagine p115 with couscous p102
Fruit fool p133

Wednesday

Breakfast
Date porridge p98 with pear slices p130

Lunch
Home-made hummus p111 with breadsticks/cucumber

Dinner
Fruity chicken p112 with mashed sweet potato
Canned peaches with semolina pudding p134

Thursday

Breakfast
Yogurt with strawberry slices p130

Lunch
Cod, pea, and potato p72

Dinner
Beef with prunes p116 with cooked spinach and rice
Stewed apple and cranberries p129

Friday

Breakfast
Mango and vanilla p97

Lunch
Lentil and spinach dhal p128 with rice

Dinner
Creamy salmon and pasta p121
Rice pudding p135 with added dried fruit

Saturday

Breakfast
Wheat biscuit with fruit/milk p70

Lunch
Sweet potato, barley, and leek soup p102 with cheesy polenta twigs p108

Dinner
Cauliflower cheese p125
Papaya fingers p131

Sunday

Breakfast
Millet and banana porridge p68

Lunch
Cheesy tomato risotto p124

Dinner
Creamy vegetable korma p126 with rice
Creamy apricot dessert p129

Other ideas this week
Spicy banana toast p100 • Cheesy polenta twigs p108 with roasted Mediterranean vegetable dip p107 • Normandy pork p113 with mashed sweet potato and steamed green beans • Greek baked fish p120 with cooked spinach • Apple and pear fingers p130

day-by-day meal planner
Week 4

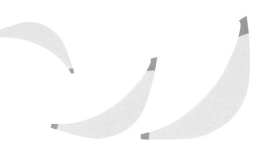

Monday

Breakfast
Date porridge p98 and mango slices p131

Lunch
Flaked salmon p106 with avocado dip p105

Dinner
Creamy vegetarian mince p126 with rice
Berries with chocolate dipping sauce p135

Tuesday

Breakfast
Toast and cream cheese p100 with pear slices p130

Lunch
Butternut squash risotto p122

Dinner
Tofu with spinach and rice p127
Creamy apricot dessert p129

Wednesday

Breakfast
Fromage frais and mashed berries

Lunch
Hard-boiled egg with buttered toast p69 and pepper fingers

Dinner
Greek baked fish p120 with mashed potato
Stewed apple and cranberries p129

Thursday

Breakfast
Spicy banana toast p100

Lunch
Tofu and avocado dip p108 with steamed carrot p118–19

Dinner
Baby's first lamb tagine p115 with couscous p102 and cooked spinach
Chocolate rice pudding p135

Friday

Breakfast
Mango and vanilla p97

Lunch
Coconut lentil dhal p128 with rice

Dinner
Italian tomato and tuna mash p120
Banana with chocolate dipping sauce p135

Saturday

Breakfast
French toast with strawberry slices p98

Lunch
Sweet potato, barley, and leek soup p102 with cheesy polenta twigs p108

Dinner
Chicken Provençale p112 with pasta shapes
Semolina pudding p134 and apricot purée p60

Sunday

Breakfast
Apple and raspberries p97

Lunch
Yummy veggie sauce with pasta p122 and grated cheese

Dinner
Beef with prunes p116 with broccoli and rice
Fromage frais with fruit

Other ideas this week Blueberry breakfast p97 • Toast and peanut butter p101 • Lentil and spinach dhal p128 • Steamed vegetable fingers pp118–19 with home-made hummus dip p111 • Garden vegetable risotto p127 • Herby lamb with vegetables p114 • Fruit fool p133

day-by-day meal planner
Week

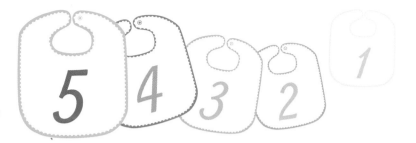

5 4 3 2 1

Monday

Breakfast
Wheat biscuit p70 and banana slices

Lunch
Carrot and lentil soup p103 with bread

Dinner
Salmon and sweet potato cakes p121 with yogurt and green beans
Fromage frais with fruit

Tuesday

Breakfast
French toast with fruit p98

Lunch
Tuna dip p105 with breadsticks/ raw or steamed vegetables pp118–19

Dinner
Creamy vegetable korma p126 with rice
Fruits of the forest iced yogurt p133

Wednesday

Breakfast
Millet porridge p68 with stewed fruit p129

Lunch
Yummy veggie sauce with pasta p122 and grated cheese

Dinner
Normandy Pork p113 with mashed potato and broccoli
Yogurt with fruit purée p96

Thursday

Breakfast
Banana and kiwi p97

Lunch
Scrambled egg p99 with toast and raw or steamed vegetables pp118–19

Dinner
Creamy vegetarian mince p126 with couscous p102 and carrots
Fruit fool p133

Friday

Breakfast
Raspberry porridge p99

Lunch
Italian tomato and tuna mash p120

Dinner
Pork with pineapple p114 and steamed courgette p118
Lemony ricotta pudding p134

Saturday

Breakfast
Yogurt with strawberry slices p130

Lunch
Avocado dip p105 with steamed vegetables pp118–19 and breadsticks

Dinner
Cheesy tomato risotto p124 and green beans
Apply plums p129

Sunday

Breakfast
Banana oat porridge p68

Lunch
Mini lamb and mint balls p109 with avocado dip p105

Dinner
Creamy salmon and pasta p121
Soft pear slices p130

Other ideas this week Mango and vanilla breakfast p97 • Cheese scones p104 with cottage cheese dip p107 • Sweet potato, barley, and leek soup p102 • Beef ragu p115 with pasta shapes and broccoli • Chicken and mushroom casserole p113 with mashed potato and green beans • Chocolate rice pudding p135

day-by-day meal planner
Week 6

Monday

Breakfast
Blueberry and pear p97

Lunch
Carrot and lentil soup p103 with bread

Dinner
Pork with pineapple p114 with rice and broccoli
Ground rice pudding p134 with mashed berries

Tuesday

Breakfast
Fromage frais with banana slices

Lunch
Coconut lentil dhal p128 with rice

Dinner
Herby lamb with vegetables p114 and couscous p102
Stewed apple and raisins p129

Wednesday

Breakfast
Toast and cream cheese p100 and halved grapes

Lunch
Scrambled egg p99 with toast/soft tomato pieces

Dinner
Cheesy tomato risotto p124 and sweetcorn
Creamy apricot dessert p129

Thursday

Breakfast
Yogurt with whole raspberries

Lunch
Cauliflower cheese p125 and bread fingers

Dinner
Salmon and sweet potato cakes p121 with avocado dip p105 and green beans
Semolina pudding p134 with fruit

Friday

Breakfast
Bircher muesli p98

Lunch
Avocado dip p105 with dippers pp104–110

Dinner
Beef with prunes p116 with potatoes and broccoli
Yogurt with fruit purée p96

Saturday

Breakfast
Scrambled egg p99 with toast

Lunch
Sweet potato, barley, and leek soup p102

Dinner
Chicken Provençale p112 with mashed potato
Fruit fool p133

Sunday

Breakfast
Spicy banana toast p100

Lunch
Italian tomato and tuna mash p120 with cooked spinach

Dinner
Macaroni cheese p125 and steamed vegetables pp118–19
Mango lolly p132

Other ideas this week   Date porridge p98 • Toast and peanut butter p101 • Broccoli cheese p125 with bread fingers
• Baby falafel p110 with home-made hummus p111 • Baby's first vegetable curry p123 with rice
• Avocado slices with toast fingers • Fruity chicken p112 with mashed potato • Apply plums p129

day-by-day meal planner Week 7

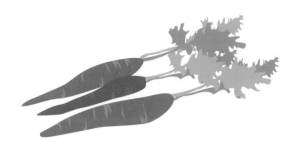

Monday

Breakfast
Bircher muesli p98

Lunch
Cauliflower cheese p125 and bread fingers

Dinner
Herby lamb with vegetables p114 and couscous p102
Berries with chocolate dipping sauce p135

Tuesday

Breakfast
Mango and vanilla p97

Lunch
Home-made hummus p111 with pitta bread and pepper fingers

Dinner
Beef ragu p115 with pasta and courgettes
Mango lolly p132

Wednesday

Breakfast
Raspberry porridge p99

Lunch
Italian tomato and tuna mash p120 with cooked spinach

Dinner
Butternut squash risotto p122 with green beans
Banana custard p133

Thursday

Breakfast
Toast and cream cheese p100 and halved grapes

Lunch
Carrot and lentil soup p103 with cheese scones p104

Dinner
Baby's first vegetable curry p123 with chapatti fingers
Fromage frais with fruit

Friday

Breakfast
Wheat biscuit with milk p70/mashed blueberries

Lunch
Cottage cheese dip p107 with rice cakes

Dinner
Greek baked fish p120 with mashed potato and courgettes
Soft pear slices p130

Saturday

Breakfast
Stewed fruit p129 and yogurt with spoon of muesli

Lunch
Baby falafel p110 with roasted Mediterranean vegetable dip p107

Dinner
Normandy Pork p113 with broccoli and baby pasta
Fruit fool p133

Sunday

Breakfast
Bircher muesli p98

Lunch
Broccoli cheese p125 with bread fingers

Dinner
Lentil and spinach dhal p128 with rice
Yogurt with fruit purée p96

Other ideas this week — Spicy plum and banana breakfast p96 • Flaked fish p106 with avocado dip p105 • Sweet potatoes with sardines and peas p117 • Chicken Provençale p112 with mashed potatoes and broccoli florets • Macaroni cheese p125 • Stewed apple and cranberries p129

day-by-day meal planner
Week

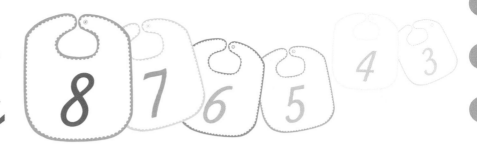

8 7 6 5 4 3

Monday

Breakfast
Spicy banana toast p100

Lunch
Penne pasta with roasted Mediterranean vegetable dip p107

Dinner
Herby lamb with vegetables p114 and mashed potatoes
Yogurt with fruit purée p96

Tuesday

Breakfast
Raspberry porridge p99

Lunch
Tuna dip p105 on toast with halved cherry tomatoes

Dinner
Beef and onion casserole p116 with mashed root vegetables
Chocolate rice pudding p135 and orange pieces

Wednesday

Breakfast
Bircher muesli p98

Lunch
Creamy vegetable korma p126 with rice

Dinner
Greek baked fish p120 with mashed potatoes and green beans
Mango lolly p132

Thursday

Breakfast
Apricot porridge p68

Lunch
Italian tomato and tuna mash p120

Dinner
Pork with pineapple p114 with rice and cooked spinach
Fruits of the forest iced yogurt p133

Friday

Breakfast
Blueberry and pear p97

Lunch
Mini lamb and mint balls p109 with roasted Mediterranean vegetable dip p107

Dinner
Garden vegetable risotto p127
Papaya fingers p131

Saturday

Breakfast
Toast and cream cheese p100 and canned peach slices

Lunch
Tofu and avocado dip p108 with raw or steamed vegetables p118–19 or breadsticks

Dinner
Chicken Provençale p112 with mashed vegetables
Yogurt with stewed fruit p129

Sunday

Breakfast
Mixed spice drop scones p99

Lunch
Flaked salmon p106 with avocado dip p105 and bread and butter

Dinner
Beef with prunes p116 with cooked spinach and rice
Semolina pudding p134 and apricot purée p60

Other ideas this week
Strawberry fromage frais breakfast p96 • Toast fingers p69 with cottage cheese dip p107 • Carrot and lentil soup p103 with cheese scones p104 • Cauliflower cheese p125 with toast fingers p69 • Tofu with spinach and rice p127 • Peach and nectarine slices p131

day-by-day meal planner
Week 9

By the end of stage 2, your baby has experienced many new tastes and is learning to chew more challenging textures.

Monday

Breakfast
Yogurt with mango slices p131

Lunch
Tuna dip p105 on toast with halved cherry tomatoes

Dinner
Creamy vegetable korma p126 with rice
Fruit fool p133

Tuesday

Breakfast
Oat porridge with banana slices p98

Lunch
Baby falafel p110 with yogurt and raw or steamed carrot sticks pp118–19

Dinner
Beef ragu p115 with pasta shapes and broccoli
Mango slices p131

Wednesday

Breakfast
Mixed spice drop scones p99

Lunch
Carrot and lentil soup p103 with cheese scones p104

Dinner
Fruity chicken p112 with mashed potato and cooked spinach
Yogurt with mashed fruit

Thursday

Breakfast
Bircher muesli p98

Lunch
Little sausage and apple balls p106 with apple purée dip p59 and bread

Dinner
Cauliflower or broccoli cheese p125
Sliced pear or apple p130

Friday

Breakfast
Wheat biscuit with milk p70 and raisins

Lunch
Garden vegetable risotto p127

Dinner
Salmon and sweet potato cakes p121 with avocado dip p105
Strawberry or kiwi slices p130

Saturday

Breakfast
Strawberry slices p130 and fromage frais

Lunch
Roasted Mediterranean vegetable dip p107 with pasta

Dinner
Chicken Provençale p112 with rice
Banana with chocolate dipping sauce p135

Sunday

Breakfast
Spicy plum and banana p96

Lunch
Salmon and sweet potato cakes p121 with broccoli

Dinner
Herby lamb with vegetables p114 and couscous p102
Stewed apple and raisins p129

Other ideas this week Apple and raspberry breakfast p97 • Hard-boiled egg and buttered toast p69 • Sweet potatoes with sardines and peas p117 • Ratatouille p124 • Chicken and mushroom casserole p113 • Semolina pudding p134 with stewed fruit p129

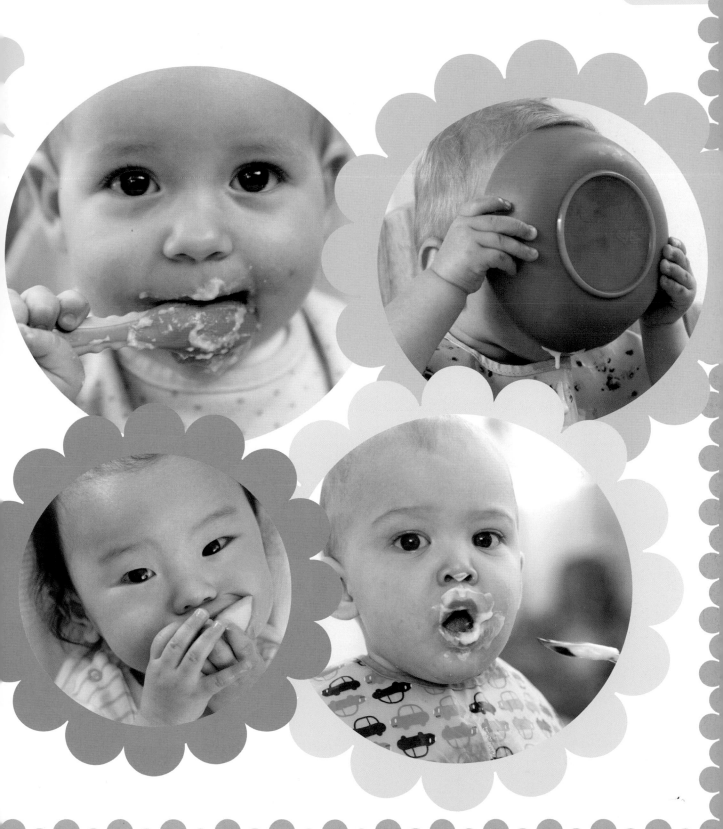

Tailor-made days

As you become more practised and confident about preparing nutritious meals for your baby, you may find you have days when you want to tailor the meal plans to suit your own lifestyle. We all have times when the meals we cook are shaped by how demanding our day is, or which ingredients we have to hand. On some days, especially those when your baby wakes up fretful or clingy, time to cook is in short supply; whereas on others, time spent in the kitchen is soothing and satisfying. As you move into stage 3 of weaning, the top 10s that follow can help you tailor the odd day in the meal plans to suit your requirements.

Meals for leisurely days

Slow-cooking dishes or ones that involve a bit more preparation are perfect for at-home days when you've more time on your hands. The longer cooking times for some of these meals also free up time for you to spend with your baby and get household chores done while dinner takes care of itself.

Slowly stewed meat is infused with flavours and deliciously tender, making it easy for your baby to chew.

1 Sweet potato, barley and leek soup p102

2 Butternut/pumpkin and tomato soup p180

3 Normandy pork p113

4 Baby's first lamb tagine p115

5 Beef and onion casserole p116

6 Beef with prunes p116

7 Cheesy tomato risotto p124

8 Ratatouille p124

9 Garden vegetable risotto p127

10 Vegetarian shepherd's pie p189

Certain foods benefit nutritionally from longer cooking times. Tomatoes release more of the protective antioxidant lycopene during the cooking process.

And puddings:

· Rice pudding p135

· Baked stuffed apple p190

· Pear and raisin oat crumble p193

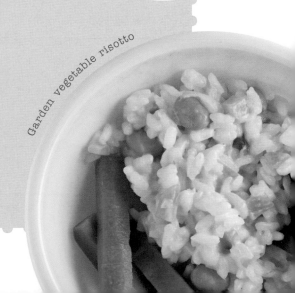

Garden vegetable risotto

Meals for busy days

The recipes here are spot on for days when you've been out and about and have little time left for cooking. Quick to rustle up, each dish has nutritional value, too. If you know certain days will be a little hectic, buy core fresh ingredients, such as fish or chicken, ahead for the fridge or freezer to reach for when needed.

1 Pesto, tomato, and mozzarella pizza p178

2 Pea and mint soup p181

3 Fruity chicken p112

4 Chicken and pasta with creamy sauce p183

5 Pork with pineapple p114

6 Cheesy mash with fish and peas p117

7 Greek baked fish p120

8 Cauliflower/broccoli cheese p125

9 Creamy vegetarian mince p126

10 Creamy avocado pasta p188

And puddings:

· Creamy apricot dessert p129

· Fresh fruit pp130–31

· Exotic fruit salad p191

· Passion fruit and mango dessert p191

Shorter cooking times preserve more of the essential vitamins B and C, making quick-cook dishes convenient and healthy.

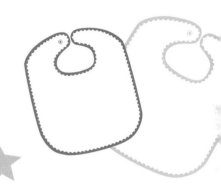

Commercially frozen vegetables often provide as much vitamin C as their fresh equivalents, and are a godsend on days when you're pressed for time.

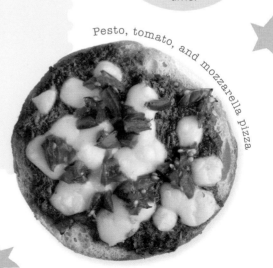

Pesto, tomato, and mozzarella pizza

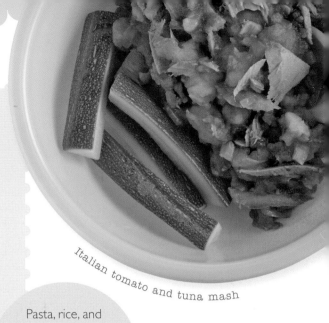

Storecupboard recipes

For days when fresh supplies are running low and you can't get to the shops, a well-stocked cupboard and some core fridge items offer some great meal solutions. The recipes below provide some delicious meals and lighter bites that can be easily prepared from storecupboard basics.

1 Cheese scones p104

2 Polenta twigs p108 with tuna dip p105

3 Scrambled eggs p99

4 Sardines/beans on toast p173

5 Italian tomato and tuna mash p120

6 Macaroni cheese p125

7 Tofu with spinach and rice p127

8 Coconut lentil dhal p128

9 Cowboy beans with cornmeal topping p188

10 Fruity couscous with peanut sauce p189

And puddings:

· Fruits of the forest iced yogurt p133

· Semolina pudding p134

· Bread and butter pudding p194

· Baked egg custard p195

Italian tomato and tuna mash

Pasta, rice, and couscous are core staples for your storecupboard, providing a starchy base for many dishes.

Canned beans provide protein and are super convenient: most require heating just briefly before adding to dishes, avoiding the more lengthy soaking process needed for dried beans.

Fruits of the forest iced yogurt

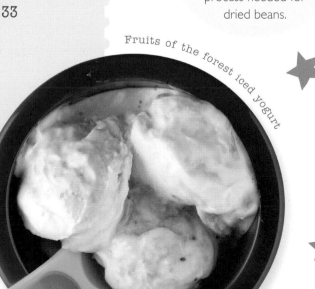

Economy dishes

As food prices rise, we are all a bit more conscious of what goes in the weekly food shop. The good news is that being economical doesn't have to equal less healthy eating. For weeks when you want to cut down a little on more costly meat and fish dishes, recipes using pulses, hearty soups, and simple pasta dishes all provide filling, nutritious, and cost-effective meals.

1 Carrot and lentil soup p103

2 Baked potato with Mexican beans p177

3 Mushroom and onion pizza p178

4 Leek and potato soup p180

5 Italian tomato and tuna mash p120

6 Butternut squash risotto p122

7 Baby's first vegetable curry p123

8 Macaroni cheese p125

9 Lentil and spinach dhal p128

10 Vegetarian shepherd's pie p189

And puddings:

· Apply plums p129

· Banana custard p133

· Semolina p134

· Baked spiced peach p190

Baked potatoes are nutritious, versatile – being the perfect base for a variety of delicious toppings – and a great source of energy.

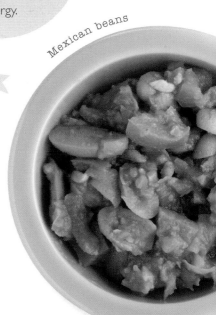
Mexican beans

Vegetables and fruits are cheaper in season, when they also tend to be more nutritious.

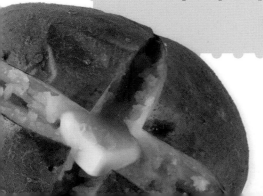

Ways with *purées*

Purées are a great introduction to solids, getting your baby used to new tastes and textures. As weaning progresses and your baby's repertoire of foods expands, purées continue to be a useful way to include fruits and vegetables in her diet, whether as an addition to breakfasts and puddings or a topping for toast.

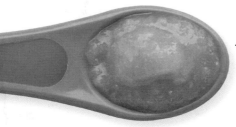

Apricot yogurt breakfast

Mix 1 tablespoon of apricot purée (p60) with 1 tablespoon of full-fat yogurt.

Spicy peach breakfast

Mix a pinch of cinnamon with 1 tablespoon of peach purée (p61), and stir into 1 tablespoon of full-fat yogurt or fromage frais.

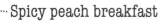

Plain yogurt

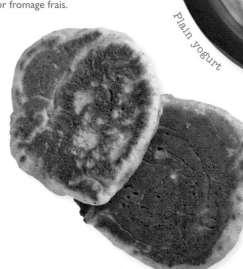

Spicy peach breakfast

Spicy plum and banana breakfast

Stew 2 small ripe plums, which you have washed and quartered, in 1 tbsp water until they are soft. Blend until smooth. Mash half a small banana and stir in the plum purée along with a pinch of mixed spice.

Strawberry fromage frais

Wash and hull 2 medium ripe strawberries. Mash well with a fork until smooth, and stir into 1 heaped tablespoon of full-fat yogurt or fromage frais.

With drop scones!

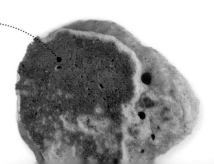

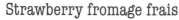

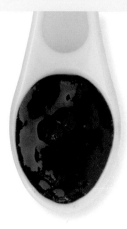

Blueberry breakfast

Mix 1 tablespoon of blueberry purée (p60) with 1 tablespoon of full-fat yogurt or fromage frais.

Apple and raspberry breakfast

Take 3–4 fresh or defrosted raspberries and mash into 1 tablespoon of apple purée (p59).

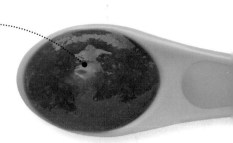

Blueberry and pear breakfast

Mix 1 tablespoon of blueberry purée (p60) with 1 tablespoon of pear purée (p59).

With toast

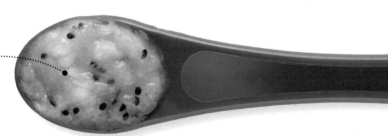

With yogurt or fromage frais

Banana and kiwi breakfast

Peel and halve a ripe kiwi fruit, removing the white core, and mash well with a fork. Mash half a small banana and mix with the kiwi.

Mango and vanilla breakfast

Mix 1 tablespoon of mango purée (p59) with 2 drops of vanilla extract and combine with 1 tablespoon of full-fat yogurt or fromage frais.

With cereals

Porridge

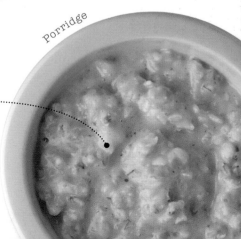

Bircher muesli

This Swiss-derived muesli uses grated apples and juice and is soaked overnight in the fridge, which softens all the ingredients. It makes a delicious and healthy start to the day, so make a batch for both you and your baby.

 5 mins | Soaking time: overnight | 1 baby and 1 adult portion

ingredients

1 heaped tbsp **rolled oats**
1 medium **eating apple**,
 peeled, cored, and grated
3 tbsp **orange juice**
3 heaped tbsp **full-fat plain yogurt**
pinch of **mixed spice**
raisins (optional)

method

1 Blend the oats and process until fine. Place in a bowl.

2 Add all the other ingredients except the raisins and mix well. Cover with cling film and refrigerate overnight.

3 Stir a few raisins into your portion, if you like, but do not add any to your baby's portion until she is used to chewing more solid food.

✱**Serve** *with mashed blueberries or a few slices of banana.*
✱**Store** *in the refrigerator in an airtight container for up to 48 hours.*
✱**Variations:** *Add 1 dessertspoon of ground almonds or desiccated coconut in step 1. As your baby becomes more used to chewing, omit step 1.*

French toast with fruit

French toast, or "eggy bread", makes a nutritious start to the day. This recipe uses a slice of brioche, which is soft and enriched with milk and eggs. Serve with any fruit: slices of kiwi or soft pear, or blueberries. Your baby only needs half an egg, so this makes enough for two.

5 mins | 1 baby and 1 adult portion

4–6 mins

ingredients

1 **egg**
1–2 tsp **butter** or **olive oil**

2–3 small slices of **brioche loaf**
fruit of choice, to serve

method

1 Beat the egg in a shallow dish or plate.

2 Heat the butter or oil in a non-stick frying pan. Dip a slice of brioche into the beaten egg and quickly turn it over with a fork or tongs to coat the other side.

3 Fry for a minute on each side until lightly browned.

4 Cool a little and cut into bite-sized pieces for your baby. Serve with fruit.

✱ *Not suitable for storing.*

Basic oat porridge

Porridge oats, sometimes called rolled or flaked oats, cook more quickly than traditional oatmeal, and provide soluble fibre, which has many health benefits.

1 min | 2–3 mins | 1 portion

ingredients

30g (1oz) **porridge oats**

150ml (5fl oz) **whole milk**

method

1 Place the oats and milk in a small saucepan and heat, stirring continuously.

2 When the mixture thickens, remove from the heat. Cool to body temperature and serve.

✱**Microwave version:** *Mix the oats and milk in a microwaveable bowl and cook on high for 30 seconds (800W oven). Stir and cook for another 10 seconds. (The timing will vary according to the power of your oven.) Once thickened, remove and cool.*

✱ **Variations:** *You can add 15g (½oz) of dried, semi-dried or fresh dates. Dates provide natural sweetness as well as dietary fibre. If using dried chopped dates, you may need to soak them in hot water for 10 minutes before use, to soften them. If using fresh dates, peel off the skin, remove the stone, and then chop. Similarly, if using semi-dried dates, remove the stone and chop.*

Raspberry porridge

A lovely pink porridge, this is quick to make and will go down quickly as well.

 1 min   2–3 mins 1 portion

ingredients

30g (1 oz) **porridge oats**
150 ml (5fl oz) **whole milk**

4–5 **raspberries**, fresh, or frozen and defrosted

method

1 Place the oats and milk in a small saucepan and heat, stirring continuously.

2 When the mixture thickens, add the raspberries, and stir in

well so that the fruit breaks up.

3 Remove from the heat and cool to body temperature before serving.

✱ Microwave version: *Mix oats and milk in a microwaveable bowl and cook on high for 30 seconds (800W oven). Stir and cook for 10 seconds. (Timing varies according to the oven's power.) Once thickened, remove, add the raspberries, and cool.*

Scrambled egg

An easy, nutritious breakfast, scrambled eggs provide protein, iron, and vitamins A and D. Depending on your baby's appetite, you may need to help her eat this. Or use two larger eggs and have some, too.

 2 mins   2 mins 1–2 portions

ingredients

1 **egg**
2 tbsp **whole milk**

1 tsp **olive spread**

method

1 In a small bowl, beat together the egg and milk.

2 Heat the spread in a small saucepan and when melted stir in the egg mixture.

3 Cook over a low heat until the egg just thickens.

4 Spoon into a bowl and allow to cool to body temperature.

5 Serve with toast fingers.

Mixed spice drop scones

English drop scones aren't dissimilar to American pancakes, but usually are smaller and made with fresh milk, not buttermilk. A handy snack, these are also a good finger food addition to fruit at breakfast.

 5 mins   10–15 mins   16 drop scones

ingredients

100ml (3½fl oz) **whole milk**
1 **egg**
75g (2½oz) **self-raising flour**
50g (1¾oz) **wholemeal flour**

1 tbsp **maple syrup**, or 2 tsp, **sugar**
¼ tsp **mixed spice**
1 tbsp **vegetable oil**, for greasing

method

1 Place a griddle or non-stick frying pan over a medium–high heat.

2 Meanwhile, blend all the ingredients except the oil until you have a thick batter.

3 Brush the pan or griddle lightly with oil

and spoon a few dessertspoonfuls of batter into the pan to make individual pancakes. Cook 1 minute on one side, then carefully turn over to cook the other side. When fully cooked, remove from the pan and cool slightly before serving or storing.

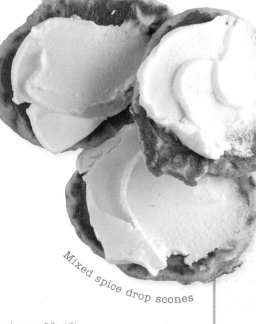

Mixed spice drop scones

✱ **Serve** *with cream cheese, butter or spread. These can also be served with a fruit purée (see pp59–62).*
✱ **Store** *in the cupboard in an airtight container for up to 24 hours, or freeze when cool.*
✱ **Variations:** *Once your baby can chew more efficiently, try adding a handful of raisins to the mixture after blending.*

Ways with *toast*

Toast makes an easy breakfast once your baby can self-feed, and by the end of this stage, she will be quite adept at coping with finger foods. It's important not to rely on buttered toast alone, as your baby needs protein (eggs, dairy or meat) and fruit, too.

Spicy banana toast

This fruity addition to your baby's toast fingers provides essential vitamins and slow-release energy to keep her going through the morning.

ingredients

½ slice of **white bread**
butter or
monounsaturated
spread

pinch of **cinnamon**
few slices of **banana**

method

1 Toast the bread lightly and spread the butter over it.

2 Sprinkle over the cinnamon and cut into bite-sized pieces.

3 Place the banana slices on top and serve.

Toast and cream cheese

Cream cheese provides less protein than cottage or curd cheese, but is fine to use occasionally. Your baby doesn't need the low-fat varieties of cream cheese, so if you are buying for the family, make sure hers is full-fat.

method

1 Any type of bread without hard seeds or grains is fine – try white, wholemeal or brioche bread. Toast the bread lightly and spread about 1 tablespoon of cream or curd cheese per slice. A portion for a baby of 7–9 months is ½–1 small slice.

2 Serve with sliced strawberries or kiwi fruit. For an older baby, try raw red pepper pieces or halved, seeded cherry tomatoes.

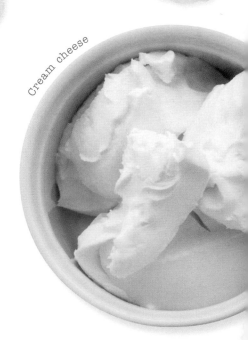

Cream cheese

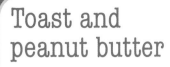

Toast and peanut butter

Use low-salt and low-sugar peanut butter, and a smooth variety as crunchy ones can cause choking. If allergies run in the family, consult your doctor before giving your baby peanut butter.

method

1 You can use white or wholemeal bread, or try with pitta bread. Toast the bread lightly and spread approximately 1 tablespoon of peanut butter a slice. A portion for a 7–9 month-old baby is ½–1 small slice.

2 Serve with sliced bananas or halved blueberries. For an older baby, serve with raw cucumber pieces.

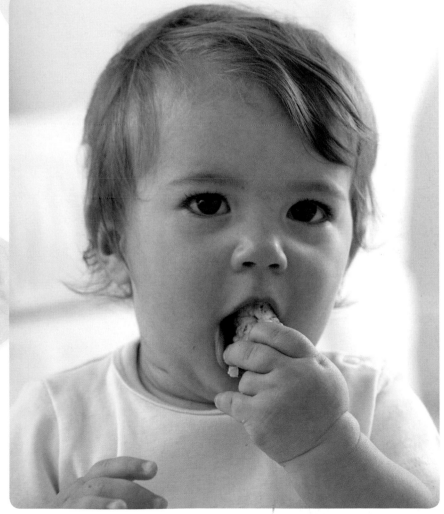

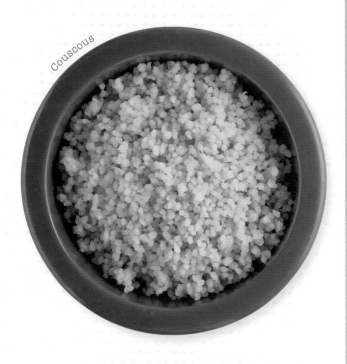

Couscous

This very easy starchy accompaniment is enjoyed by babies as it is soft, and by parents as it doesn't require much effort to make! It is available wholewheat or plain, and with large or small grains; this recipe uses the most commonly found small-grained plain type.

 1 min   1 baby portion

5 mins

ingredients

10g (¼oz) or 1 tbsp **couscous**

method

1 Place the couscous in a small ramekin or bowl and pour over 2 tablespoons of boiling water. Stir and allow to stand for 5 minutes.

2 Fluff with a fork and serve.

✳ **Variations:** *Add 1 teaspoon of olive oil with the water. For citrus couscous, use 1 tablespoon of boiling water and 1 tablespoon of freshly squeezed orange juice.*

Sweet potato, barley, and leek soup

Sweet potatoes make delicious soups, as well as providing a huge boost of vitamin A. Adults, babies, and children will enjoy this mild sweet soup, and it is worth making a double batch so you can freeze it for a cold day, when it makes a welcoming warm lunch. Fresh stock improves the flavour, but don't add salted stock to your baby's food.

 15 mins   40–45 mins   3–4 baby and 3 generous adult portions

ingredients

1 tbsp **olive oil**
175g (6oz) **leek**, sliced finely
150g (5½oz) **carrots**, peeled and diced
200g (7oz) **sweet potatoes**, peeled and diced
750ml (1¼ pints) **salt-free vegetable or chicken stock**
50g (1¾oz) **pearl barley**
3 **bay leaves**
a few **parsley stalks** (optional)
salt and **pepper**, to taste

method

1 Heat the oil in a non-stick saucepan and gently fry the leeks for 5 minutes, softening, but not browning it. Add the carrots and sweet potatoes, stir, and cover. Sweat the vegetables for another 5 minutes.

2 Add the stock, barley, bay leaves, and parsley. Bring to the boil, stir, cover, and simmer for 30–35 minutes, stirring occasionally.

3 Remove the bay leaves and the parsley. Add the parsley to the mixture to be blended.

4 Allow to cool slightly, then blend half the soup, and mix with the remaining soup.

5 Remove your baby's portion, blend further, if needed, and serve at body temperature. Season your portion, adding salt and pepper as needed, and serve.

✳ **Serve** *with Cheese scones (see p104), bread or rolls.*
✳ **Refrigerate** *in an airtight container for up to 24 hours or freeze when cool.*
✳ **Variations:** *A large onion can be used instead of the leek.*

Carrot and lentil soup

This simple soup uses wholesome inexpensive ingredients that both you and your baby can enjoy together. Offer a couple of tablespoons of soup in her bowl and allow her to enjoy dipping a few fingers of toast or bread into it. You can then spoon-feed more to her as required.

 5 mins   25–30 mins   2 baby and 2 generous adult portions ❄

ingredients

1 tbsp **vegetable oil**, for frying
100g (3½oz) or 1 small **leek**, finely sliced
250g (9oz) **carrots**, peeled, and diced
150g (5½oz) **celeriac** or **swede**, peeled and diced
50g (1¾oz) **split red lentils**
750ml (1¼pints) **salt-free vegetable or chicken stock**
1 **bay leaf**
salt and **black pepper**, to taste
pinch of **grated nutmeg**, to serve

method

1 Heat the oil in a large non-stick saucepan and gently fry the leeks for 3–4 minutes until soft. Add the carrots and celeriac, stir, cover, and sweat for 5 minutes without browning the vegetables.

2 Stir in the lentils, stock, and bay leaf and bring to the boil, stirring occasionally.

3 Cover, reduce the heat, and simmer for 15–20 minutes, or until the vegetables are tender and the lentils have become soft. Take off the heat and remove the bay leaf.

4 Remove a portion for your baby and allow to cool a little before processing to a suitable texture. Pour into your baby's bowl and allow to cool to body temperature before serving.

5 Meanwhile, for your portion adjust the seasoning in the remainder of the soup, adding a little salt and black pepper, as desired. If you like a chunky soup, process half the soup until smooth and mix with the rest of it in the pan. If you prefer a smoother soup, blend the whole portion.

6 Pour into a bowl and grate over a pinch of nutmeg.

✱ **Serve** *with pieces of wholemeal or white toast.*

✱ **Refrigerate** *in an airtight container for up to 24 hours or freeze when cool.*

✱ **Variations:** *Celery can be used, but as it can be fibrous, it is recommended that the soup be puréed well to avoid stringy parts remaining.*

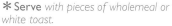
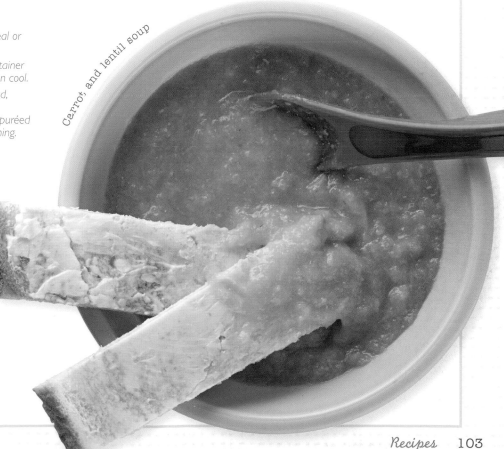

Dips and *dippers*

For babies who like to self-feed, home-made dips can be an easy way of providing protein and vegetables, and there are lots of interesting things to serve them with. As well as breadsticks, rice cakes, and oatcakes, try the dippers suggested here. Dips are best made and served fresh as most don't freeze well.

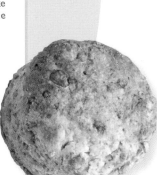

Cheese scones

Little cheese scones can be made in a jiffy and taste great with soup, as well as being handy for breakfast or a quick snack. Use strong Cheddar so you can taste the cheese.

 10 mins   12–15 mins   10–12 small scones

ingredients

- 125g (4½oz) **wholemeal flour**
- 125g (4½oz) **plain white flour**, plus extra for dusting
- 3 tsp **baking powder**
- 25g (scant 1oz) **full-fat butter** or **spread**
- 50g (1¾oz) **Cheddar cheese**, grated
- 150ml (5fl oz) **whole milk**, plus extra for brushing

method

1 Preheat the oven to 200°C (400°F/Gas 6).

2 Sieve the flours and baking powder into a bowl, adding back any bran that remains. Rub the butter or spread into the flour and stir in the grated cheese.

3 Using a small palette or round-ended knife, stir the milk into the dry ingredients until you have a soft, but not sticky, mixture. Press the mixture into a ball. Sprinkle a little flour on a clean board or work surface and roll out, or gently press the dough to around 1.5cm (½in) thick.

4 Place a baking sheet in the hot oven for a couple of minutes.

5 Using 4–5cm (1½–2in) cutters, stamp out scones until the dough is used up, gently re-rolling unused dough.

6 Carefully place the scones on the hot baking tray and brush the tops with a little milk. Bake for 12–15 minutes, or until the scones are risen and golden. Cool and serve fresh.

✳ *Serve with creamy cheese or monounsaturated spread. These are also delicious with soup, or dips and vegetable batons.*

✳ *These are best eaten on the day they are made. Refrigerate in an airtight container for up to 24 hours or freeze when cool.*

✳ **Variations:** *Replace the wholemeal flour with white flour.*

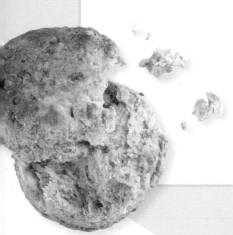

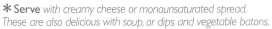

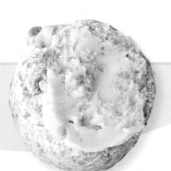

Avocado dip

Avocados are a good source of protective vitamin E as well as healthy monounsaturated fats. Simply mash with a little lemon juice to prevent browning, and add in other ingredients as you wish to introduce new flavours and textures.

🕐 5 mins   🚫   ◔ 1 baby and 1 adult portion

ingredients

1 ripe **avocado**, halved and stone removed
juice of ½ **lemon**

Optional additions to make guacamole:

1 ripe **tomato**, skinned and deseeded, finely chopped
1 **spring onion**, trimmed and finely chopped (once your baby can chew properly)
few drops **Tabasco sauce**

method

1 Scoop out the avocado flesh from the shell and mash until smooth with the lemon juice.

2 Serve at once, or add other ingredients to make guacamole.

✱ **Serve** *with Flaked fish (see p106), steamed vegetable batons (raw for older babies), baby breadsticks or pieces of pitta bread. Alternatively, use as a filling for sandwiches.*

✱ *Not suitable for storing.*

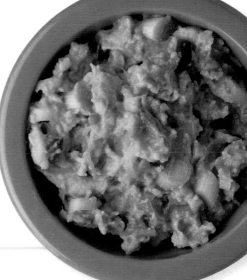
Avocado dip

Tuna dip

Tuna is a storecupboard essential, and is often well accepted by babies. However, the canning process destroys most of the important omega 3 fatty acids, so don't rely exclusively on tuna as an oily fish; try salmon and sardines in your baby's diet, too. This dip is simple to make and is delicious with lots of different dippers.

🕐 5 mins   🚫   ◔ 2 baby and 2 adult portions

ingredients

70g (2½oz), or ½ can, **tuna** in oil, drained
50g (1¾oz) **full-fat cream cheese**
10g (¼oz) or 1 dessertspoon **tomato purée**
finely grated zest of half small **lemon**
½ tsp finely chopped **dill**

method

1 Process all the ingredients until smooth.

2 Spoon into a small container(s). Cover and chill until required.

✱ **Serve** *with baby breadsticks, pieces of cucumber or pepper, or cooked carrot and green beans.*

Little sausage and apple balls

Using premium-quality sausages and fresh apple, these little balls are ideal for small hands to hold for self-feeding. They are quick to make and freeze well. Pork is a great source of vitamin B1 (thiamine).

 5 mins 15–20 mins 6–7 small balls

ingredients

65g (2oz) or 1 premium quality **sausage**, skinned
50g (1¾oz) or ½ medium **apple**, peeled and coarsely grated
20g (¾oz) fresh **breadcrumbs**

method

1 Preheat the oven to 190°C (375°F/Gas 5).

2 Process all the ingredients, or mix together with a fork until well combined. Shape into balls around the size of an unshelled walnut.

3 Place on a greased baking sheet and bake in the oven for 15–20 minutes, or until the centre is piping hot and cooked through. Allow to cool before serving.

✳**Serve** *with a dip, such as Roasted Mediterranean vegetable dip (see opposite) or Avocado dip (see p105).*

✳**Refrigerate** *in an airtight container for up to 48 hours, or freeze when cool.*

✳**Variations:** *Instead of baking in the oven, fry in 1 tablespoon of vegetable oil, browning on all sides. Drain on kitchen paper.*

Flaked fish

A white fish such as cod or a thick piece of salmon has large flakes that a baby can hold and eat. These are great for dipping in tomato salsa or other dips. Choose a thick piece of fish fillet, weighing around 100g (3½oz), and run your finger over the flesh to check for any bones, removing any you find. Bake, steam or microwave until the fish is opaque. When you press it, it should gently break into flakes. Cool a little, remove the skin, and then give your baby a few flakes to enjoy.

method

Bake
Bake at 180°C (350°F/Gas 4) for 15 minutes.

or

Steam
Wrap in foil or baking parchment and steam for 8–10 minutes.

or

Microwave
Microwave on high for 3–5 minutes depending on the power of the oven.

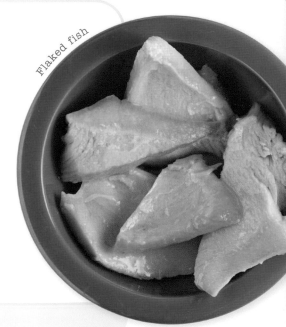
Flaked fish

Roasted Mediterranean vegetable dip

Rich in vitamins C and A, this sweet dip is great for dipping vegetables or baby breadsticks into. Alternatively, it can be used as a sandwich filling.

 5 mins   25–30 mins   1 baby and 1 adult portion

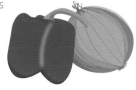

ingredients

- 1 **red pepper**, cut into large chunks
- 6 ripe **cherry tomatoes**, halved
- 1 small **red onion**, peeled and chopped
- 1–2 tbsp **olive oil**
- 5 large **basil leaves**, torn into 2 or 3 pieces
- 100g (3½oz) **mascarpone cheese**
- 2 tsp **lemon juice**

method

1 Preheat the oven to 200°C (400°F/Gas 6).

2 Place the pepper, tomatoes, and onion in a roasting tin, drizzle over the oil, and roast in the oven for 25–30 minutes, or until the vegetables are soft.

✳ Serve *with Cheesy polenta twigs (see p108) or Mini lamb and mint balls (see p109).*

3 Allow to cool for a few minutes, then blend until smooth. Add the basil, mascarpone, and lemon juice, and pulse lightly to mix. Chill until required.

Roasted Mediterranean vegetable dip

Cottage cheese dip

Richer in protein and calcium than cream cheese or fromage frais, cottage cheese blends to a smooth consistency, making simple dips and easy sandwich spreads for your baby.

 5 mins   1 min   2 baby and 1 adult portion

ingredients

- 100g (3½oz), or 2 ripe medium **tomatoes**
- **full-fat plain cottage cheese**
- 25g (scant 1oz) **Cheddar cheese**, grated
- 2 tsp **chives**, washed and snipped

method

1 Skin the tomatoes by scoring the flesh with a cross at the base and covering with boiling water for 20 seconds. Remove, peel off the skin, and cut the tomatoes into four, then scoop out the seeds.

2 Blend all the ingredients until smooth. Serve at once, or chill for later use.

✳Serve *with baby rice cakes or breadsticks, or steamed vegetable batons.*

Cheesy polenta twigs

Gluten-free polenta or cornmeal can be shaped and baked as a finger food. As it freezes well, it is worth making a batch and keeping some for later as it is a wheat-free alternative to breadsticks.

🕐 2 mins ♨ 5–10 mins ◔ 10–12 twigs ❄

ingredients

40g (1½oz) quick-cook **polenta** or **cornmeal**

40g (1½oz) **hard cheese**, such as Leicester or Cheddar, grated

method

1 Preheat the oven to 190°C (375°F/Gas 5).

2 Place the polenta and 110ml (3¾fl oz) water in a saucepan and bring to the boil, stirring constantly until the mixture thickens and leaves the sides of the pan. Remove from the heat and stir in the cheese.

3 When cool enough, break off pieces of the dough and shape into "twigs" 4–5cm (1½–2in) in length and as thick as your finger. Bake for 15 minutes to harden, cool, and store.

✳ **Serve** *with dips, or as an alternative to pieces of toast or breadsticks.*

✳ **Refrigerate** *in an airtight container for up to 48 hours or freeze when cool.*

Tofu and avocado dip

Tofu is a bland soya bean curd that is an amazingly good source of calcium, so it is ideal if your baby can't tolerate dairy products. It also provides iron, which the vitamin C-rich tomatoes in the recipe ensure can be easily absorbed.

🕐 5 mins ♨ 1 min ◔ 2 baby and 1 adult portion

ingredients

1 ripe medium **tomato**
1 ripe small or ½ medium **avocado**

60g (2oz) **tofu**
1 tsp **lemon** or **lime juice**

method

1 Skin the tomato by scoring the flesh with a cross at the base and covering with boiling water for 20 seconds. Remove, peel off the skin, and cut the tomato into four, then scoop out the tomato seeds.

2 Halve the avocado and remove the stone. Scoop out the flesh.

3 Blend all the ingredients until smooth and serve at once, or chill for up to 24 hours.

✳ **Serve** *with steamed vegetables, cooked pasta shapes or baby breadsticks.*

✳ **Best served** *on the day of cooking. Refrigerate in an airtight container for up to 24 hours.*

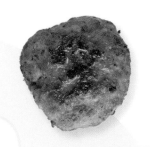

Mini lamb and mint balls

These tiny meat balls are a good source of iron and ideal for baby-led weaning. Blend the ingredients together well to eliminate lumpy bits that your baby might struggle to chew.

🕐 5 mins   🔥 12–15 mins   🕐 15 mini balls   ❄️

ingredients

½ small **onion**, roughly chopped
½ small slice of **bread**, torn into a few pieces
150g (5½oz) **lamb mince**
1 tsp chopped **mint**
a little **flour**
1–2 tbsp **vegetable oil**

method

1 Process the onion, bread, lamb, and mint until fine and well blended. Check for any large lumps and process again if needed.

2 Tip the mixture onto a clean board or plate. If the mixture is sticky, add a little flour before dividing into 15 parts. Roll each part into a neat ball.

3 When they are all prepared, heat the oil in a non-stick frying pan and fry gently over a low to medium heat, browning on all sides. Drain on kitchen paper, cool, and serve 1 or 2 per meal, heated to piping hot, then allowed to cool to body temperature.

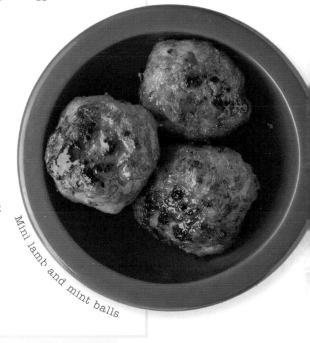

Mini lamb and mint balls

✱ **Serve** with a dip, such as Roasted Mediterranean vegetable dip (see p107) or tzatziki.

✱ **Refrigerate** in an airtight container for up to 24 hours or freeze when cool.

✱ **Variations:** Use any minced meat, but beef and lamb provide more iron than turkey or chicken. Add garlic or a little grated lemon zest.

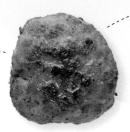
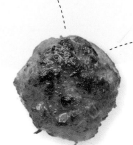
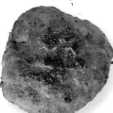
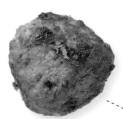
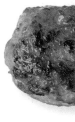

Baby falafel

An easy food for your self-feeding baby to manage, and a great one to take out and about, baby falafels are simple to make and a reasonable source of vegetable-based iron.

 10 mins   15 mins   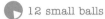 12 small balls

ingredients

- 2 tbsp **vegetable oil**, plus extra for frying
- 1 medium **onion**, finely chopped
- 1 **garlic clove**, crushed
- 1 tsp ground **cumin**
- 1 tbsp chopped **coriander**
- 1 tbsp chopped **parsley**
- 400g (14oz) can **chickpeas** in water, rinsed and drained
- 1 **egg**, beaten
- **wheat flour** or **gram flour** (chickpea flour), for shaping

method

1 Heat the oil in a frying pan and gently fry the onion and garlic until softened, but not browned. Stir in the cumin and fresh herbs and remove from the heat.

2 Process the chickpeas until smooth.

3 Add the cooked onion mixture and 1 tablespoon of the egg to the chickpeas and process again, adding more egg, if needed, to make a soft but not too sticky mixture. Shape the mixture into loose balls, using flour if it feels too sticky.

4 Heat 3–4 tablespoons of oil in a frying pan and gently fry the balls in batches for around 10 minutes, turning occasionally, until they are golden brown on all sides. Drain on kitchen paper and serve warm.

✱ **Serve** *with Spicy peanut dip (see opposite), plain yogurt, and couscous (see p102).*

✱ **Refrigerate** *in an airtight container for up to 48 hours or freeze when cool.*

✱ **Variation:** *For an older baby or child, mash or process the chickpeas and stir in the cooked onion mixture, rather than processing it all.*

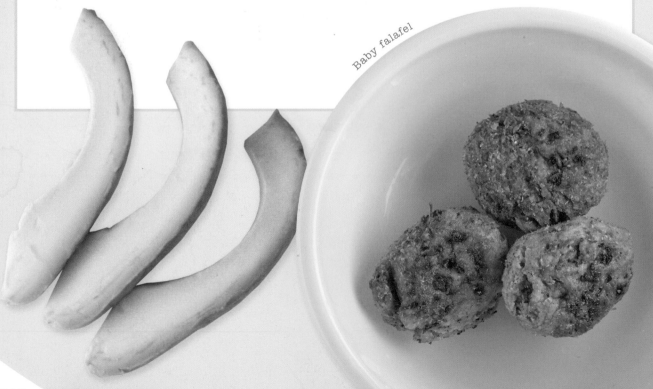

Baby falafel

Home-made hummus

Using a can of chickpeas is the easiest way to make hummus. If you prefer to soak and boil chickpeas, you'll need around 100g (3½oz) dried beans. Tahini is made from crushed sesame seeds, which are a good source of calcium. You can add the crushed garlic to your portion once you've removed your baby's portion if you prefer.

 5 mins 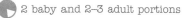 2 baby and 2–3 adult portions

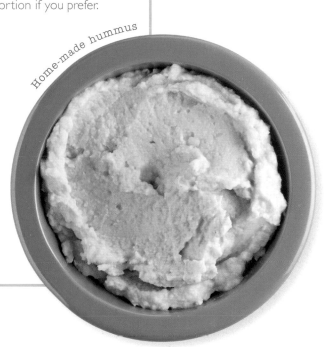

Home-made hummus

ingredients

400g (14oz) can **chickpeas** in water, rinsed and drained
1 small **garlic clove**, crushed (optional)
1 heaped tbsp **tahini** (sesame seed paste)
1 tbsp **lemon juice**
2 tbsp **extra virgin olive oil**

method

1 Blend all the ingredients until smooth. If the mixture is a little stiff, add 1 tablespoon of water at a time to loosen.

2 Remove your baby's portion and refrigerate the rest. Season your portion to taste.

✷ **Serve** *with pieces of pitta bread or vegetables.*
✷ **Refrigerate** *in an airtight container for up to 48 hours.*
✷ **Variations:** *There are many ways to adjust the flavour for yourself and your baby once she is used to this basic version. Try adding a few sun-dried tomatoes or finely grated lemon zest.*

Spicy peanut dip

Served warm or at room temperature, this dip is great with the Mini lamb and mint balls (see p109), or served with vegetable sticks for dunking. Peanuts are rich in protein and vitamins E and B3. If there are allergies in the family, consult your doctor before giving your baby peanuts.

 5 mins 2 mins 2 baby and 2 adult portions

ingredients

2 **spring onions**, washed, trimmed, and roughly sliced
60ml (2fl oz) **whole milk**, plus extra if needed
½ tsp **garam masala** or **ground cumin**
1 tsp chopped **coriander**
100g (3½oz) **smooth peanut butter**, low-/no sugar or salt

method

1 Place the onions, milk, garam masala or ground cumin, and coriander in a small saucepan and heat gently to soften the onions.

2 Cool slightly and blend with the peanut butter to make a smooth dip, adding more milk, if needed.

✷ **Serve** *with Mini lamb and mint balls (see p109) or Baby falafel (see opposite).*

Chicken Provençale

Full of Mediterranean favourites, Chicken Provençale is a bumper source of vitamin C and is enjoyed by babies and parents alike. It freezes well so make a batch when peppers and courgettes are plentiful to use as your baby grows.

 7–8 mins   20–25 mins   5–6 baby portions or 1 adult and 2 baby portions   ❄

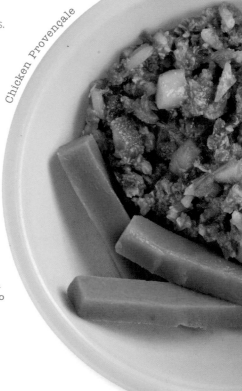

Chicken Provençale

ingredients

1 tbsp **olive oil**
1 small **onion**, finely chopped
120g (4oz) or 1 **skinless chicken thigh fillet**, cut into 2cm (¾in) pieces
½ **red pepper**, quartered and finely chopped
½ medium **courgette**, quartered lengthwise and sliced
200g (7oz) can chopped **tomatoes**
6 **basil leaves**, washed and torn
1 tbsp **couscous** or **rice**, cooked

method

1 Heat the oil in a non-stick saucepan and gently fry the onion for 2–3 minutes before adding the chicken. Continue to fry for 2–3 minutes until the chicken is lightly cooked on each side.

2 Stir in the pepper, courgette, and tomatoes. Stir, cover, and bring to a simmer. Reduce the heat and cook gently for 15–20 minutes, or until the vegetables and chicken are tender.

3 Add the basil leaves in the last 5 minutes of cooking and, if the mixture is looking dry, add 1 tablespoon of water.

4 When cooked, remove your baby's portion and adjust the texture. Serve with a tablespoon of cous cous or rice mashed into the mixture.

✳ Serve *with pieces of cooked carrot alongside.*

✳ Refrigerate *in an airtight container for up to 48 hours or freeze when cool.*

✳ Variations: *Add a slice or two of aubergine instead of or as well as the courgette.*

Fruity chicken

Rich in vitamin A, mango makes a delicious addition to this chicken casserole. Using darker thigh meat provides more iron than if you use the whiter breast meat. The raisins also top up the iron quota.

 5 mins   20 mins   6 baby portions or 2 baby and 1 adult portion   ❄

ingredients

1 tbsp **vegetable oil**
1 small **onion**, finely chopped
100g (3½oz) **skinless chicken thigh fillet** cut into 2cm (¾in pieces)
½ tsp **ground cumin**
30g (1oz) **raisins**
150g (5½oz) **mango**, cut into cubes (see p131)

method

1 Heat the oil in a non-stick saucepan and lightly fry the onion and chicken for 4–5 minutes without browning.

2 Stir in the cumin, raisins, and 150ml (5fl oz) water, and bring to a simmer. Stir, reduce the heat, and cook over a gentle heat, checking occasionally, for 10 minutes.

3 Add the mango cubes and cook for 5–6 minutes, or until very tender.

4 Cool slightly, remove your baby's portion, and adjust the texture by processing a little before serving.

✳ Serve *with green vegetables.*

✳ Refrigerate *in an airtight container for up to 24 hours or freeze when cool.*

Chicken and mushroom casserole

Chicken is a good source of protein. As with Fruity chicken (see opposite), the darker thigh meat supplies more iron than the white breast. Mushrooms provide iron, too, which the body absorbs more easily than from other plant foods.

 5 mins   20–25 mins   5–6 baby portions or 1–2 baby and 1 adult portion

ingredients

1 tbsp **vegetable oil**
160g (5¾oz) **skinless chicken thigh fillets**, cut into 2–3cm (¾–1in) pieces
90–100g (3¼–3½oz) or 1 small **courgette**, sliced
60g (2oz) **closed cap/button mushrooms**, sliced
1 tsp chopped **thyme**

method

1 Heat the oil in a non-stick saucepan and fry the chicken until sealed all over. Stir in the courgettes, mushrooms, and thyme with 150ml (5fl oz) water.

2 Bring to a simmer, stir, and cover. Reduce the heat and cook for 15–20 minutes, or until the vegetables are tender and the chicken is cooked through. Remove from the heat and allow to cool slightly.

3 If you are eating the casserole too, remove your baby's portion and blend to the necessary texture. Season your portion with black pepper, and if you like, a little salt.

✳ **Serve** *with mashed potatoes or wedges of boiled potatoes, carrots or squash, and green vegetables.*

✳ **Refrigerate** *in an airtight container for up to 24 hours or freeze in individual labelled containers when cool.*

✳ **Variations:** *You can add 1 small finely chopped onion in step 1.*

Normandy pork

Made with pork and apples, this dish is bound to be a hit with your baby. For speed use minced pork, but if the oven is on, you can use any stewing pork, cooking it slowly to tenderize it and then processing.

 5 mins   30–35 mins   3–4 baby portions

ingredients

1 tbsp **vegetable oil**
½ small **onion**, finely chopped
100g (3½oz) **lean pork mince**
1 medium **apple**, peeled, cored, and grated
150ml (5fl oz) **cloudy apple juice**, plus more if needed
½ tsp chopped **sage**

method

1 Heat the oil in a non-stick saucepan and gently fry the onion and mince together, using a spoon to break up the mince. Stir in the apple, juice, and sage, and cover.

2 Simmer gently for 20–25 minutes, or until the mixture is tender, stirring and adding more juice, if needed.

3 Process to a suitable consistency.

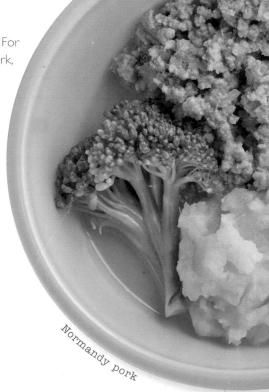

Normandy pork

✳ **Serve** *with mashed potato or steamed potato pieces and a green vegetable.*

✳ **Refrigerate** *in an airtight container for up to 24 hours or freeze on the day of cooking when cool.*

Pork with pineapple

Your baby will enjoy this simple sweet and sour style of pork. It uses a can of pineapple pieces in juice, which are softer than fresh pineapple and available cheaply all the year round.

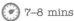 7–8 mins   30 mins   5–6 baby portions or 2 baby and 1 adult portion

ingredients

1 tbsp **vegetable oil**
150g (5½oz) **lean pork mince**
2 small **celery sticks**, finely chopped
½ small **onion**, finely chopped
227g (8oz) can of **pineapple** pieces in juice
1 tbsp **tomato purée**
1 tsp **wine vinegar**

method

1 Heat the oil in a non-stick saucepan and gently fry the mince, breaking it up with a spoon as it cooks.

2 Add the celery and onion and continue cooking over a medium heat for 2–3 minutes to fry the vegetables.

3 Drain the pineapple and reserve the juice in a measuring jug. Add the pineapple pieces to the saucepan.

4 Add the purée and vinegar to the pineapple juice and add water until the jug measures 150ml (5fl oz) of liquid. Add to the pan.

5 Bring to a simmer, stir, cover, and cook gently for 20 minutes, or until the mixture is tender.

6 Remove your baby's portion and process to a suitable consistency before serving. Season your portion with a little soy sauce, if desired, and serve.

* **Serve** *with mashed plain boiled rice and steamed green vegetables as finger food.*
* **Refrigerate** *in an airtight container for up to 24 hours or freeze on the day of cooking when cool.*
* **Variations:** *Use canned apricots in juice instead of pineapple.*

Herby lamb with vegetables

This simple recipe uses lamb mince, and if you're making the Mini lamb and mint balls (see p109), it's a great one to cook at the same time, as one 500g (1lb 2oz) pack of lamb mince will provide you and your baby with several meals.

 7–8 mins   30–35 mins   4–6 baby and 3 adult portions

ingredients

350g (12oz) **lean lamb mince**
120g (4¼oz) or 1 medium **onion**, finely chopped
120g (4¼oz) or 1 large **carrot**, peeled and finely diced
200g (7oz) **butternut squash**, peeled and finely diced
1 tbsp chopped fresh, or ½ tbsp dried, **mint**
1 tbsp chopped **thyme**
1 tbsp **tomato purée**

method

1 Place the mince and onion in a non-stick saucepan and heat gently, allowing the fat from the mince to fry the onions. Break the mince up with a wooden spoon as you continue to cook for 5–7 minutes, or until the mince is lightly browned.

2 Add the carrot, squash, herbs, and tomato purée and stir well.

3 Pour in 300ml (10fl oz) water and bring to a simmer. Stir, cover, reduce the heat, and simmer for another 25–30 minutes, or until the vegetables are tender and the mince is cooked through completely.

4 Take off the heat and remove your baby's portions – approximately 1 heaped tablespoon of mixture per portion.

5 Blend your baby's portion to a suitable texture, perhaps reserving some soft pieces of carrot or squash for her to eat with her fingers.

6 For your portion, adjust the seasoning if you need to, and serve with rice, potatoes or couscous (see below), and a green vegetable.

* **Serve** *every tablespoon of lamb and vegetables with 1 heaped tablespoon of cooked rice or couscous, blending if necessary, or mashed potato.*
* **Refrigerate** *in an airtight container for up to 24 hours or freeze.*

Baby's first lamb tagine

In this slow-cooked dish, dried fruit and meat provide a sweet iron-rich combination for your baby. Serve with couscous (see p102) for a real Moroccan flavour.

 5 mins   80–90 mins   2 6 baby portions or 2 baby and 1 adult portion

ingredients

150g (5½oz) **lamb**, such as neck fillet or steak, cut into 1.5–2cm (½–¾in) cubes
1 small **onion**, finely chopped
1 **garlic clove**, crushed
100g (3½oz) **dried fruit**, such as prunes and apricots, halved
½ tsp **ground cumin**
½ tsp **ground coriander**
2 tbsp **tomato purée**

method

1 Preheat the oven to 170°C (325°F/Gas 3).

2 Place all the ingredients with 200ml (7fl oz) water in a small casserole dish, stir well, cover, and cook in the oven for 1 hour, checking and stirring occasionally, adding more water if necessary.

3 Return and cook for a further 20–30 minutes, or until the lamb is tender. Cool slightly and remove your baby's portion. Process to a suitable consistency and serve.

*Serve *with couscous and cooked pieces of green beans or courgette.*

*Refrigerate *in an airtight container for up to 24 hours or freeze on the same day when cool.*

* Variations: *Swap half of the dried fruit for raisins.*

Beef ragu

A beef ragu is a family staple that can be used to make lasagne, served with pasta as a Bolognese sauce or used as a meaty dip for babies who like to self-feed. Beef is rich in iron and zinc, and choosing lean mince will cut down on saturated fats.

 10 mins   35–40 mins   2 2 baby and 2 adult portions

ingredients

1 tbsp **vegetable oil**
½ small **onion**, finely chopped
1 **garlic clove**, crushed
250g (9oz) **lean steak mince**

½ **red pepper**, finely chopped
200g (7oz) can chopped **tomatoes**
2 tbsp **tomato purée**
½ tsp **thyme** or **oregano**

method

1 Heat the oil in a non-stick saucepan and gently fry the onion, garlic, and mince, breaking up the meat with a wooden spoon for 5 minutes until the mince is separated. Add the red pepper and continue frying, stirring frequently, until it is soft and the meat has browned.

2 Add the tomatoes, tomato purée, and herbs with 50ml (1¾fl oz) water and bring to a simmer. Stir, cover, and cook for 25–30 minutes, or until the sauce has thickened; add water if needed.

3 Remove from the heat, process to a suitable texture for your baby, if needed, and serve at body temperature.

*Serve *with pasta shapes, broccoli florets, and pieces of carrot.*

* Refrigerate *for 48 hours or freeze on day of making when cool.*

* Variations: *You can use lamb or pork mince if you prefer, or even try it with a vegetarian mince.*

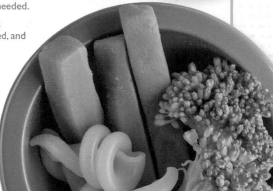
Beef ragu

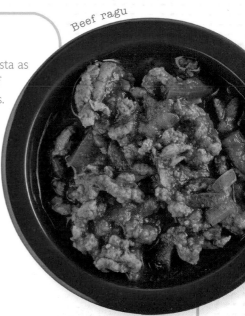

Beef and onion casserole

Slowly braised meat becomes tender and easier to eat, which is ideal for babies who are learning to chew. Using beef ensures your baby has a good supply of easily absorbed iron. This is a casserole or stew at its most basic, which you can adapt by adding different vegetables, herbs or meats.

 10 mins    1½–2 hours   3 baby and 1 adult portion

ingredients

2 tbsp **vegetable oil**

100g (3½oz) or 1 medium **onion**, finely chopped

400g (14oz) **lean braising steak**, cut into 2–3cm (¾–1in) cubes

250g (9oz) or 2 large **carrots**, peeled and cut into 1cm (½in) thick slices

1 **bay leaf**

1 tbsp **flour (wheat or cornflour)**

method

1 Preheat the oven to 170°C (325°F/Gas 3).

2 Heat the oil in an ovenproof pan and gently fry the onion for 2–3 minutes. Add the beef to the pan and lightly brown on all sides, stirring frequently while browning.

3 Stir in the carrots, 400ml (14fl oz) water, and add the bay leaf. Bring to a simmer, cover, and place in the oven for 1 hour.

4 Remove from the oven. Mix the flour with 2 tablespoons of water and a little of the cooking juice, and stir this into the casserole.

5 Cover and return to the oven for 30–45 minutes, or until the beef is very tender and separates easily when cut with a knife.

6 Remove the bay leaf, take out your baby's portion, and allow to cool slightly. Blend until the meat is a soft consistency and serve or cool before freezing.

✳ **Serve** *with mashed potato and broccoli florets.*

✳ **Refrigerate** *in an airtight container for up to 48 hours or freeze when cool.*

✳ **Variations:** *This recipe can be made with stewing lamb. You can use parsnips, swede, and celeriac instead of, or as well as, the carrots. Remove some carrots before puréeing the meat, and then roughly mash or chop these into the mixture.*

Beef with prunes

A slowly cooked stew with prunes makes a delicious main meal for you and your baby and also freezes well. The addition of a little tomato paste provides vitamin C to help with iron absorption from the beef.

 5 mins   80–90 mins   6 baby portions or 2 baby and 1 adult portion

ingredients

200g (7oz) **lean braising steak**, cut into 1–2cm (½–¾in) cubes

1 small **onion**, finely chopped

50g (1¾oz) ready-to-eat **prunes**, halved

¼ tsp **cinnamon** (optional)

1 tbsp **tomato purée**

method

1 Preheat the oven to 170°C (325°F/Gas 3).

2 Place all the ingredients with 250ml (9fl oz) water in a small casserole dish and cover.

3 Cook in the oven for 1 hour, stirring occasionally. Check and add more water if needed. Return and cook for a further 20–30 minutes, or until the beef is tender.

4 Cool slightly and remove your baby's portion. Process to a suitable consistency and serve.

✳ **Serve** *with mashed potato, sweet potato or couscous, and steamed green vegetables.*

✳ **Refrigerate** *in an airtight container for up to 48 hours or freeze when cool.*

Sweet potatoes with sardines and peas

Canned sardines are an excellent source of many important nutrients including iron, zinc, calcium, and vitamin B12, as well as providing omega 3 fatty acids. Although not always popular, they're an inexpensive "superfood", so it is worth persevering. Buy in water, oil or tomato sauce, and drain well before mashing with a fork or blending.

 5 mins   10–15 mins   3–4 baby portions ❄

ingredients

120–150g (4¼–5½oz) or
  1 small **sweet potato**,
  peeled and cut into
  small cubes
50g (1¾oz) **frozen peas**,
defrosted
1–2 tbsp **water** or **milk**
35g (1oz) canned
  sardines, drained

method

1 Steam the sweet potatoes for 10–12 minutes, allow to cool a little, and mash.

2 Steam the peas for 2–3 minutes until hot through, and then purée with the water or milk.

3 Mash the fish until fine and mix with the pea purée. Stir the mixture into the mashed potato, and serve warm.

✳ Refrigerate *in an airtight container for up to 24 hours or freeze when cool.*
✳ Variations: *Pilchards are just larger sardines, and are equally nutritious.*

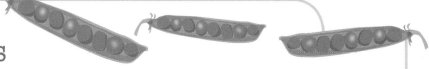

Cheesy mash with fish and peas

A yummy introduction to eating fish. Choose a sustainably sourced white fish such as pollock, cod or haddock. Even fillets can sometimes have small bones, so check for bones by running a finger over the flesh of the fish.

 10 mins   15 mins   4–6 baby portions ❄

ingredients

200g (7oz) **potatoes**,
  peeled and quartered
2 tsp **monounsaturated
  spread**, such as
  olive spread
13cm (5in) small **leek**
  (only the white part), cut
  into quarters lengthwise
  and finely sliced
60g (2oz) skinless **fillet
  of white fish**
1 **bay leaf**
150ml (5fl oz) **whole milk**
50g (1¾oz) **frozen peas**,
  defrosted
25g (scant 1oz) **hard cheese**,
  such as Cheddar, grated

method

1 Steam the potatoes until tender.

2 Meanwhile, heat the spread in a non-stick saucepan and gently fry the leek, stirring frequently, until it is just softening.

3 Add the fish, bay leaf, and milk, and bring to a simmer. Cover and poach very gently for 8–10 minutes, or until the fish is opaque and flakes easily. Take off the heat, remove the fish, and discard the bay leaf, saving the milk for blending.

4 Steam the peas until tender. Mash the potatoes, using some of the saved milk, and stir in the grated cheese.

5 Mash or roughly blend the fish and peas with a little milk to a suitable consistency. Mix with the cheesy potatoes and serve at once or chill for later use.

✳ Refrigerate *in an airtight container for up to 24 hours or freeze when cool.*
✳ Variations: *You can omit the cheese, or mash 1 tablespoon of creamy cheese into the potato instead of the milk and Cheddar.*
Adjust the texture by keeping the peas and fish as finger food, served with the mashed potato.

Vegetable finger foods

Vegetables make great finger foods, allowing your baby to participate in self-feeding as well as encouraging good dietary habits. Initially, vegetables need to be cooked lightly to soften them, but as your baby gets older, some, such as peppers and carrots, can be left raw to provide varied texture and tastes.

Steaming

Vegetables should be steamed until they are tender when pierced with a sharp knife. After steaming, leave to cool to room temperature.

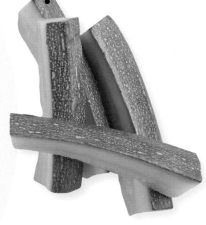

Courgettes

Choose small courgettes, trimming away the base and cutting into pieces approximately 3cm (1in) in length.

Pumpkin and squash

1 Slice off a piece weighing around 100g (3½oz).

2 Cut away the hard skin and remove any seeds.

3 Cut into pieces approximately 3cm (1in) in length.

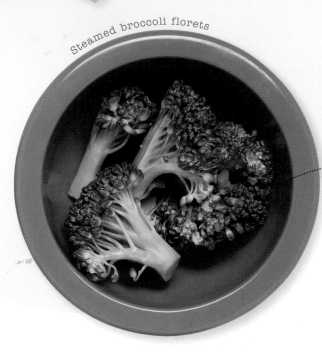

Steamed broccoli florets

Broccoli and cauliflower

Broccoli and cauliflower should be cut into small florets that your baby can hold.

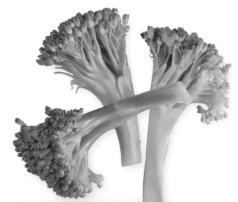

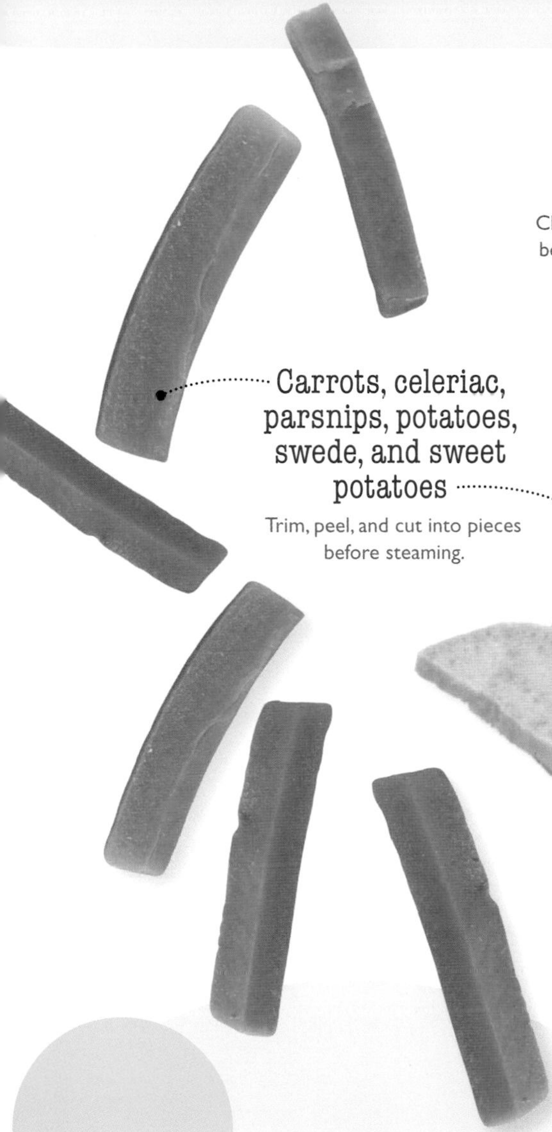

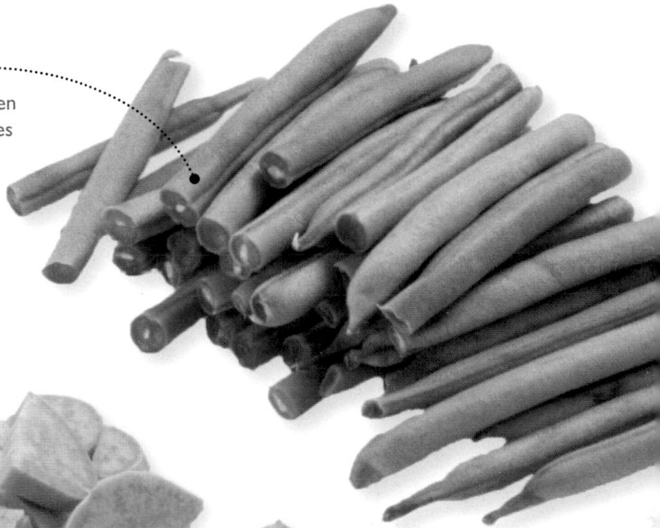

Green beans

Choose stringless round green beans, and cut into 2–3 pieces depending on their length.

Carrots, celeriac, parsnips, potatoes, swede, and sweet potatoes

Trim, peel, and cut into pieces before steaming.

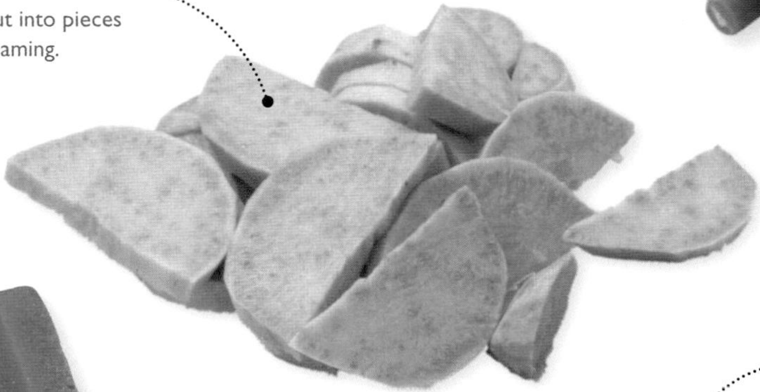

Red peppers

Wash, halve, cut away the stalk, and remove the seeds. Cut into strips about 2cm (¾in) wide and 5–6cm (2–2½in) long. Serve raw or roasted (see below).

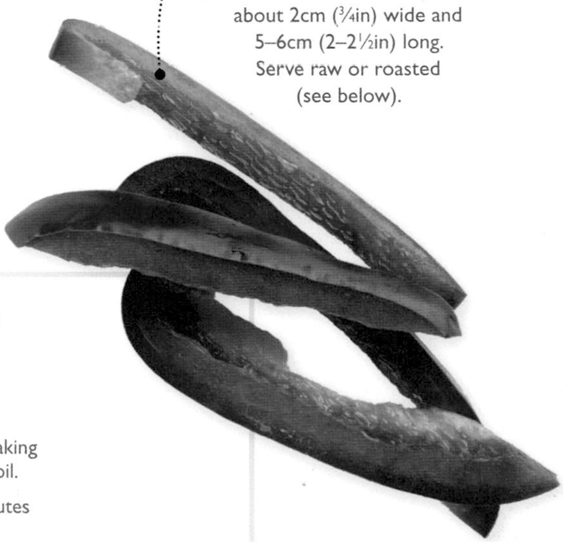

Baking or roasting

If the oven is on, it is worth roasting certain vegetables as this increases their natural sweetness.

method

1 Preheat the oven to 200°C (400°F/Gas 6).

2 Carrots, celeriac, parsnips, potatoes, swede, sweet potatoes, squash, pumpkin, and courgettes can be prepared into finger food as above.

3 Place any of these vegetables on a baking sheet and brush lightly with vegetable oil.

4 Bake for 20–25 minutes (15–20 minutes for peppers), or until the pieces of vegetables are tender.

5 Place on kitchen paper to drain off any excess oil and serve at room temperature.

Greek baked fish

Dill or small-leaved basil and olive oil provide a traditional Greek feel to this easy fish dish. Use fully ripe tomatoes and a sustainably sourced white fish of your choice. White fish provides essential protein and iodine and B vitamins, while the tomatoes provide vitamin C.

 5–7 mins   15–20 mins   4 baby portions   ✳

ingredients

2 large **plum tomatoes**,
  approximately
  100g (3½oz) each
100g (3½oz) skinless **fish fillet**
1 tsp finely chopped **dill**,
  small-leaved basil or **parsley**
1 tbsp **olive oil**

method

1 Preheat the oven to 190°C (375°F/Gas 5).

2 To skin the tomatoes, score a small cross at the base of each tomato and place in a bowl. Pour over boiling water and leave for 20 seconds. Remove and peel off the skin. Quarter the tomatoes, remove the seeds, and chop roughly.

3 Meanwhile, check the fish for bones by running your finger over the flesh.

4 Place the tomatoes at the bottom of a small ovenproof dish and place the fish on top. Sprinkle over the herbs and drizzle with oil.

5 Cover with a lid or foil and bake for 15–20 minutes, or until the fish flakes easily and is opaque.

6 Mash or blend the mixture to a suitable texture for your baby and serve immediately, or cool and freeze.

✳ Serve *with mashed potato or sweet potato, Cheesy polenta twigs (see p108) or pasta shapes.*

✳ Freeze *in individually labelled portions when cool.*

Italian tomato and tuna mash

Tomatoes, onions, herbs, and garlic are an important part of any Mediterranean diet, and they are combined here with canned tuna for protein, iron, and zinc.

 5 mins   15 mins   5–6 baby portions   ✳

ingredients

200g (7oz) **potatoes**,
  peeled and quartered
1 tbsp **vegetable oil**
½ small **onion**, finely chopped
1 small **garlic clove**,
  crushed (optional)
200g (7oz) can chopped
  tomatoes in juice
¼ tsp dried **oregano**
60g (2oz) can **tuna** in oil
  or water, drained
whole milk, if needed

method

1 Steam the potatoes until tender.

2 Meanwhile, heat the oil in a small saucepan and fry the onion and garlic, if using, until softened.

3 Stir in the tomatoes and oregano, cover, and cook over a low to medium heat for 8–10 minutes, or until the vegetables are tender. Stir in the tuna and heat through.

4 Mash the potatoes, using a little milk, if needed. Mix the potatoes and tuna together and serve at once.

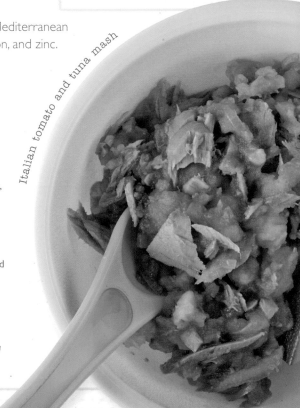

Italian tomato and tuna mash

✳ Serve *with pieces of steamed green beans, courgettes or broccoli florets.*

✳ Variations: *For babies who like to feed themselves, serve the sauce with pasta shapes, rather than mashed potato. If your baby needs a smoother consistency, purée the tuna–tomato mixture before adding to the potato.*

Salmon and sweet potato cakes

In this simple recipe, the salmon and sweet potato mixture is formed into little fish cakes, which can be hand held. The mixture can also be used without making it into fish cakes if you and your baby prefer.

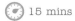 15 mins   20 mins   4 baby and 1 adult portion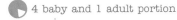

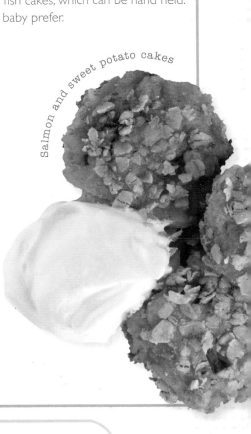

Salmon and sweet potato cakes

ingredients

250g (9oz) **sweet potatoes**, peeled and quartered
200g (7oz) skinless **salmon fillet**
1 tbsp **olive oil**
100g (3½oz), or 1 small **leek**, washed and finely chopped
75g (2½oz) **full-fat fromage frais**
zest of ½ **lemon** (optional)
50–75g (1¾–2½oz) **rolled oats**
vegetable oil, for frying

✱ Serve *with tzatziki or Roasted Mediterranean vegetable dip (see p107).*

✱ Refrigerate *in an airtight container for up to 24 hours or freeze.*

✱ Variations: *Use trout fillet. Replace the oats with crushed corn flakes and bake for 20 minutes in the oven at 190°C (375°F/Gas 5).*

method

1 Steam the sweet potatoes for 10–15 minutes, or until tender.

2 Meanwhile, run your finger over the fish to check for and remove bones. Loosely wrap the salmon in foil; place on the potatoes, or, if you have a multi-layered steamer, in another steamer, and steam for about 12 minutes.

3 Heat the oil in a frying pan; gently fry the leek until soft. When the sweet potatoes are soft, mash with the leek, fromage frais, and zest, if using.

4 Flake the fish and check for bones again, then mash into the sweet potato mixture.

5 Remove around ¼ of the mixture for your baby. Serve as is, cooling and freezing additional portions, or make into baby fish cakes as below.

6 Divide the portion into 4 small balls. Coat each ball in rolled oats. Set to one side while you make the 3–4 adult fish cakes with seasoning.

7 Heat the vegetable oil in a frying pan and fry the fish cakes for 5 minutes on each side until lightly browned. Serve warm.

Creamy salmon and pasta

Encouraging oily fish from an early age will help your baby's brain development because of the omega 3 content. This is a recipe you can do throughout the first few years, adjusting the texture as your baby is more able to chew.

 3 mins   12 mins   4–5 baby portions

ingredients

50g (1¾oz) skinless **salmon fillet**
40g (1½oz) **pasta shapes**
50g (1¾oz) small **broccoli florets**
2 tbsp **full-fat fromage frais**
whole milk, as needed

method

1 Check the salmon for bones by running your finger over the flesh. Steam or cook in the oven for around 12 minutes at 180°C (350°F/Gas 4) until the fish flakes easily.

2 Cook the pasta shapes according to the packet instructions. In the last 4 minutes, add the broccoli and continue to cook.

3 Place the salmon in a bowl and flake the fish with a fork, checking again for bones. Stir in the fromage frais. When the pasta and broccoli are softened, drain and mix with the salmon.

4 Process the mixture to an appropriate texture, adding milk as needed. Remove a portion to serve straight away, reheating if necessary. Freeze the remaining portions.

✱ Refrigerate *for 24 hours or freeze on the day of cooking.*

✱ Variations: *Use cauliflower or courgette instead of broccoli.*

Yummy veggie sauce with pasta

As soon as your baby can cope with a few lumps, you can add baby pasta shapes to sauces, or if she prefers, let her hold a soft cooked pasta bow or penne and dip it in the sauce.

 5 mins    20–25 mins   4–5 baby portions

ingredients

1 tbsp **vegetable oil**

13cm (5in) small **leek** (only the white part), cut into quarters lengthwise and finely sliced

1 small **courgette**, washed, trimmed, and finely diced

1 **garlic clove**, crushed (optional)

300g (10½ oz) can chopped **tomatoes** in juice

6 **basil leaves**, washed and roughly torn

For each portion of sauce:

15–20g (½–¾oz) cooked **pasta shapes**

1 tbsp grated **cheese**, to stir into the hot sauce, or 1–2 pieces as finger food

method

1 Heat the oil in a non-stick saucepan and gently fry the leek, courgette, and garlic, if using, for approximately 5 minutes, or until just softened.

2 Add the tomatoes and basil and bring to the boil. Stir, cover, and simmer for 15–20 minutes, or until the vegetables are soft.

3 Remove from the heat, allow to cool a little, blend to an appropriate texture, if needed, and serve with pasta shapes and cheese.

✳ Refrigerate *the sauce in an airtight container for up to 24 hours or freeze in individual labelled containers when cool.*

✳ Variations: *Use a small onion instead of leek, if you prefer.*

Butternut squash risotto

Any sort of squash or pumpkin will do for this creamy dish. You can use either special risotto rice, or short-grain rice is perfectly fine, too. This is another recipe that you can make for all the family, taking out a portion for your baby and adjusting the texture of hers.

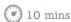 10 mins   40–45 mins   1 baby and 2 adult portions

ingredients

1 tbsp **vegetable oil**

1 medium **onion**, finely chopped

1 **garlic clove**, crushed

300g (10½ oz) **butternut squash**, peeled and cut into 5mm (¼in) cubes

150g (5½oz) **short-grain rice**

700–800ml (¼–1½ pints) **salt-free stock** or **water**

1 tbsp chopped **thyme**

For each baby portion:
1 dessertspoon **fromage frais**

For each adult portion:
grated **Parmesan cheese**
1 tbsp chopped **parsley**

method

1 Heat the oil in a non-stick sauté pan, and fry the onions over a fairly high heat for 5 minutes until softened and browning. Stir in the garlic and squash, and cook over a lower heat for 5 minutes, stirring frequently.

2 Add the rice, 150ml (5fl oz) of the stock or water, and thyme. Stir and continue cooking over a medium heat for 30–35 minutes, stirring frequently, allowing the liquid to be absorbed before adding more liquid. Continue this until all the stock has been added.

3 Remove from the heat and allow to cool slightly. Remove a portion for your baby and blend to a suitable texture, adding the fromage frais before serving. Season the remaining risotto and serve with Parmesan cheese and freshly chopped parsley.

✳ Serve *with steamed green beans or asparagus when in season.*

✳ Refrigerate *in an airtight container after cooling for up to 24 hours or freeze when cool. Defrost in the fridge overnight, or cook the frozen risotto in a covered dish at 180°C (350°F/Gas 4) for 20–30 minutes until piping hot, or in the microwave until piping hot.*

✳ Variations: *Use ricotta instead of fromage frais and add diced carrots with squash or asparagus stems in the last 10 minutes of cooking.*

Baby's first vegetable curry

A can of beans in water makes an easy and nutritious base to a vegetable curry. Use a mild curry powder so both you and your baby can enjoy this. If you like, you can season your own portion with anything spicier or hotter once her portion is served.

 5–10 mins   30–35 mins   2 baby and 2 adult portions   ❄

ingredients

2 tbsp **vegetable oil**

1 small **onion**, finely chopped

1 **garlic clove**, crushed

1 tsp **mild curry powder** (preferably salt-free)

200g (7oz) **butternut squash**, peeled and diced

200g (7oz) can or boiled **pinto** or **butter beans**

200g (7oz) can chopped **tomatoes**

For each adult portion:

Seasoning such as:

1 tsp **garam masala**

1 tbsp chopped **coriander** or **chilli sauce to taste**

method

1 Heat the oil in a saucepan, then add the onion and garlic and fry until lightly browned. Stir in the curry powder and then add the squash, beans, and tomatoes with 150ml (5fl oz) water.

2 Bring to a simmer, then reduce the heat, stir, and cover. Simmer for 20–25 minutes, stirring occasionally, and adding more water if required.

3 When the squash is tender, remove from the heat and allow to cool a little. Remove your baby's portion and adjust the texture by mashing or blending before serving. Season your portion and serve.

✳ **Serve** *with plain boiled rice, mashed to a suitable texture for your baby, or pieces of naan bread.*

✳ **Refrigerate** *in an airtight container for up to 48 hours or freeze in individually labelled portions when cool.*

✳ **Variations:** *You can use any type of beans for this recipe. Black-eyed beans provide a great source of folic acid.*

You can chop instead of mashing at step 3.

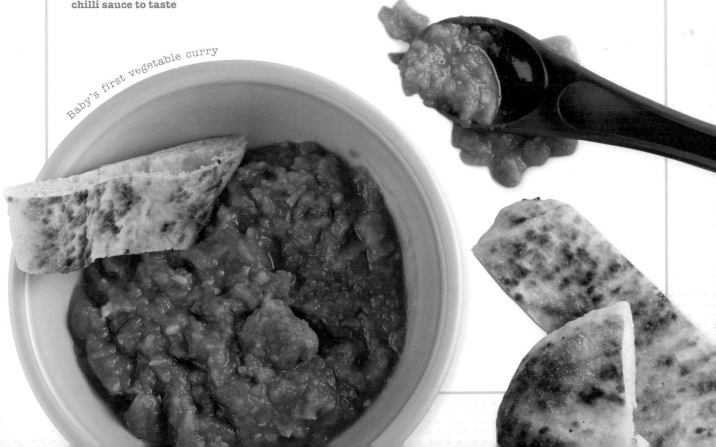

Baby's first vegetable curry

Ratatouille

Ratatouille is rich in vitamins A and C, and makes use of sun-soaked summer vegetables when they are in season. Make it for your baby from early on, adjusting the texture by mashing at first, then leaving the vegetables as cooked.

 10 mins   50–60 mins   2–3 baby and 2 adult portions ❄

ingredients

1 tbsp **olive oil**
1 small **onion**, sliced
1 **garlic clove**, crushed
¼ **red pepper**, diced roughly
¼ **green pepper**, diced roughly
2–3 slices **aubergine**, cut into 1cm (1½in) cubes

½ small **courgette**, cut into 1 cm (½in) cubes
2 medium **tomatoes**, quartered
200g (7oz) can chopped **tomatoes** in juice
½ tbsp dried oregano

method

1 Preheat the oven to 180°C (350°F/Gas 4).

2 Heat the oil in an ovenproof casserole dish and fry the onion and garlic for 3–4 minutes.

3 Add the peppers, aubergine, and courgette and stir over a medium heat for 5 minutes.

Stir in all the tomatoes and oregano, and place in the oven for 40–45 minutes, or until all the vegetables are tender.

4 Remove from the oven and cool a little. Mash or blend your baby's portion to an appropriate texture, or select soft pieces for your baby to eat as finger food.

✻ **Serve** *with couscous, rice or pasta shapes, and with a little grated cheese or mashed tofu.*
✻ **Refrigerate** *in an airtight container for up to 24 hours or freeze when cool.*

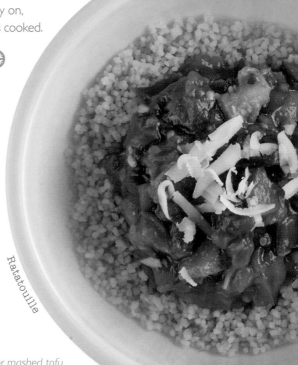

Ratatouille

Cheesy tomato risotto

A risotto is a good way of introducing your baby to grains of rice. You can cook short-grain or risotto rice until very soft, then mash if needed.

 5 mins   40 mins   6 baby portions or 2 baby and 1 adult portion

ingredients

1 tbsp **vegetable oil**
1 small **onion**, chopped
75g (2½oz) **short-grain** or **risotto rice**
300–350ml (10–12fl oz) **salt-free stock** or **water**
150g (5½oz) **tomatoes**, skinned and deseeded
2–3 **basil leaves**, washed and torn
50g (1¾oz) **Cheddar cheese**, grated

method

1 Heat the oil in a non-stick saucepan and gently cook the onion until softened. Stir in the rice and 100ml (3½fl oz) of stock or water.

2 Allow the liquid to be absorbed, stirring frequently, before adding more. Continue this until all the stock has been added.

3 Add the tomatoes and basil, and continue cooking until the rice is completely tender, adding more stock or water if needed.

4 When the risotto is cooked, stir in the cheese. Remove your baby's portion and adjust the texture if needed. Freeze additional portions.

✻ **Serve** *with steamed broccoli florets or green beans.*
✻ **Refrigerate** *in an airtight container for up to 24 hours or freeze when cool.*

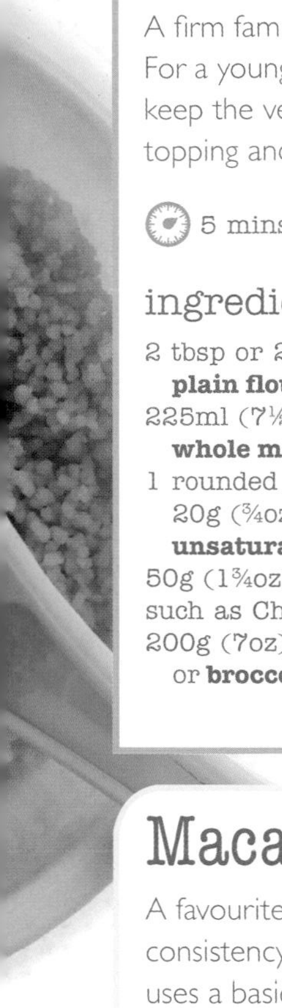

Cauliflower or broccoli cheese

A firm family favourite, this calcium-rich savoury dish can be adapted in many ways to suit all the family. For a younger baby, steam the vegetables until you can simply mash them into the sauce, and for an older baby, keep the vegetables a little firmer to encourage chewing. Also try adding a breadcrumb and grated cheese topping and baking for a few minutes for a crispy-topped variation.

5 mins | 15 mins | 3–4 baby portions

ingredients

2 tbsp or 20g (¾oz) **plain flour**
225ml (7½fl oz) **whole milk**
1 rounded tbsp or 20g (¾oz) **butter** or **unsaturated spread**
50g (1¾oz) **hard cheese**, such as Cheddar, grated
200g (7oz) **cauliflower** or **broccoli** florets

method

1 Place the flour in a saucepan off the heat and use a whisk to stir in the milk. When it is well combined, add the butter.

2 Heat gently, stirring constantly until the mixture thickens. Remove from the heat and stir in the cheese.

3 Meanwhile, steam the cauliflower or broccoli until tender. Pour the sauce over the vegetables and mash or process to a suitable consistency before serving.

* Serve *with pieces of bread and butter and halved cherry tomatoes.*
* Refrigerate *in an airtight container for up to 24 hours or freeze when cool.*

Macaroni cheese

A favourite meal for all the family, macaroni cheese is a great source of calcium. Mash or process to the correct consistency for your baby, or serve a little sauce separately and let your baby dip pasta shapes into it. This recipe uses a basic white sauce made with a fairly foolproof all-in-one method.

10 mins | 15 mins | 6 baby or 2 baby and 1 adult portion

ingredients

2 tbsp or 20g (¾oz) **plain flour**
225ml (7½fl oz) **whole milk**
1 rounded tbsp or 20g (¾oz) **butter** or **unsaturated spread**
50g (1¾oz) **hard cheese**, such as Cheddar, grated
60g (2oz) **macaroni** or **pasta shapes**

method

1 Place the flour in a saucepan off the heat and use a whisk to stir in the milk. When it is well combined, add the butter.

2 Heat gently, stirring constantly until the mixture thickens. Remove from the heat and stir in the cheese.

3 Meanwhile, cook the pasta shapes according to the packet instructions. Drain and mix into the cheese sauce.

4 Process, if needed, to a suitable consistency before serving, and freeze additional portions.

* Serve *with mashed green peas or broccoli florets.*
* Refrigerate *in an airtight container for up to 48 hours, or freeze in individual portions on the day of cooking.*
* Variations: *Add 1 tablespoon of tomato purée for a pink sauce. The sauce can also be made in a microwave oven, cooking for bursts of 30 seconds, then stopping to stir.*

Creamy vegetarian mince

A nutritious alternative to soya mince, quorn is a manufactured "mycoprotein" – a meat-free source of protein – that is high in zinc and iron.

 10 mins   25 mins 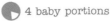 4 baby portions

ingredients

1 tbsp **vegetable oil**
½ small **onion**, finely chopped
1 **garlic clove**, crushed
  (optional)
1 small **carrot**, peeled and
  finely diced
150g (5½oz) **Quorn** or **other**
  vegetarian mince
1 tbsp **tomato purée**
150ml (5fl oz) **water**
1 tbsp chopped **parsley**

method

1 Heat the oil in a saucepan and gently fry the onion and garlic for 5 minutes until just softening.

2 Add the carrot and continue to fry for another minute or so, then stir in the quorn and tomato purée.

3 Pour in the water and bring the mixture to the boil. Then stir, cover, and simmer for

15 minutes. Check and stir occasionally, adding more water if necessary.

4 Stir in the parsley and heat through for a minute or two. Cool slightly, then blend to an appropriate consistency for your baby.

✱ **Serve** *with mashed potato and broccoli florets or green beans.*
✱ **Refrigerate** *for up to 24 hours or freeze on day of cooking when cool.*
✱ **Variations:** *Add 1–2 tsp ground coriander at stage 2.*
For extra nutrition and added creaminess, you can stir in smooth peanut butter in step 4.

Creamy vegetable korma

Coconut milk provides a creamy texture to this delicious first korma. It contains ground almonds to provide protein, but if you are not introducing nuts, replace with 2 tbsp cooked lentils or beans of your choice, adding more water if required.

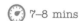 7–8 mins   15–20 mins   4–6 baby portions or 2 baby and 1 adult portion

ingredients

3–4 small **potatoes**, peeled and
  cut into cubes
1 tbsp **vegetable oil**
1 **onion**, finely chopped
1 **garlic clove**, crushed
1 tsp finely grated fresh **ginger**
1 medium **carrot**, peeled
  and diced
3–4 **broccoli florets**, cut
  into 3–4 pieces
½ tsp **turmeric**
50g (1¾oz) **ground almonds**
150ml (5fl oz) **coconut milk**

method

1 Steam the potatoes until tender. Cool slightly.

2 In a non-stick saucepan, heat the oil and gently fry the onion, garlic, and ginger for 5 minutes, adding a little water if they begin to stick to the pan.

3 Meanwhile, steam the carrot and broccoli until tender.

4 Add the turmeric to the onion mixture and stir in all the vegetables. Add the ground almonds and coconut milk, stir, and bring to a simmer.

5 Reduce the heat and continue cooking over a low heat for 5 minutes, or until the mixture is well combined and the vegetables soft.

6 Remove from the heat and cool slightly. Remove your baby's portion to blend or mash to a suitable consistency. If you are eating this yourself, adjust the seasoning to your taste.

✱ **Serve** *with a few steamed green beans as finger food.*
✱ **Refrigerate** *in an airtight container for up to 24 hours or freeze in individual labelled pots when cool.*

Garden vegetable risotto

Garden vegetables can mean all sorts of things, but carrots and beans are usually included. Here, soya or edamame beans are used alongside carrots and leek.

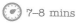 7–8 mins 35–40 mins 8 baby or 2 baby and 1 adult portion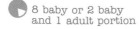

ingredients

1 tbsp **olive oil**
50g (1¾oz) or ½ small **leek**, quartered lengthwise and finely sliced
1 small **carrot**, peeled and finely diced
75g (2½oz) **short-grain** or **risotto rice**

350–400ml (12–14fl oz) **salt-free stock** or **water**
60g (2oz) frozen **soya beans**, defrosted
2 tsp chopped **thyme**
50g (1¾oz) **mascarpone cheese**

method

1 Heat the oil in a saucepan and gently fry the leek and carrot for 5–6 minutes, or until softened.

2 Add the rice and 100ml (3½fl oz) of stock or water. Allow the liquid to be absorbed, stirring frequently, before adding more. Continue this until all the liquid has been added, stirring in the beans and thyme with the last addition.

3 Continue cooking until the rice and vegetables are tender. Remove from the heat and stir in the mascarpone.

4 Remove your baby's portion, mash if necessary before serving, and freeze additional portions. If you are eating the risotto yourself, season with a little black pepper and add some Parmesan cheese.

✱ **Serve** *with additional steamed carrot batons.*

✱ **Refrigerate** *in an airtight container for up to 24 hours or freeze on the same day when cool.*

✱ **Variations**: *Use petit pois instead of soya beans.*

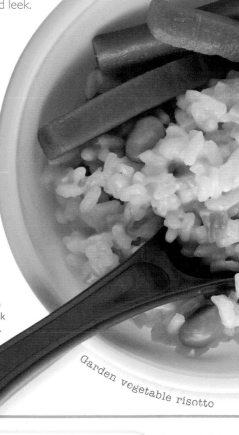

Garden vegetable risotto

Tofu with spinach and rice

Rich in calcium, tofu is a great alternative for babies who can't tolerate dairy products. Mixed with spinach and mashed rice, this dish provides your baby with a nutritious and tasty meal.

 5 mins 10 mins  4–6 baby portions

ingredients

1 tbsp **vegetable oil**
½ small **onion**, finely chopped
100g (3½oz) frozen chopped **spinach**, defrosted
150g (5½oz) **tofu**
pinch of grated **nutmeg**
100g (3½oz) cooked **long-grain white rice**

method

1 Heat the oil in a small saucepan and gently fry the onion until soft without browning.

2 Add the spinach and any defrosting juices and heat for a couple of minutes to combine, stirring constantly.

3 Remove from the heat, add the tofu, and mash well. Stir well and grate in the nutmeg.

4 For a younger baby, add the rice and blend the whole mixture. For an older baby, blend the spinach and tofu mixture, if needed, and mix with the rice, mashing as needed and serve warm.

✱ **Serve** *with steamed cauliflower or halved cherry tomatoes as finger food.*

✱ **Refrigerate** *for up to 24 hours or freeze on day of cooking when cool.*

Lentil and spinach dhal

Spinach and lentils both provide iron, although plant-based sources are not as well absorbed by the body. Vitamin C helps its absorption, so you could give your baby a drink of well-diluted unsweetened orange juice with this.

 10 mins   25–30 mins    6–8 baby or 2 baby and 2 adult portions

ingredients

1 tbsp **vegetable oil**
1 medium **onion**, finely chopped
1 **garlic clove**, crushed
125g (4½oz) spilt **red lentils**, rinsed
2 tsp **ground coriander**
2 tsp **ground cumin**
1 tbsp **tomato purée**
125g (4½oz) frozen **spinach**, thawed

method

1 Heat the oil in a non-stick saucepan and fry the onion and garlic for 4–5 minutes until lightly browned. Stir in the lentils, coriander, cumin, and 400ml (14fl oz) water, adding more if necessary.

2 Bring to a simmer, stirring occasionally, cover, and reduce the heat. Continue to cook, stirring periodically, and adding more water if the mixture is too dry.

3 When the lentils are soft, stir in the tomato purée and spinach.

4 Continue to cook for 5 minutes, or until the dhal is piping hot.

* **Serve** *with rice, pieces of chapatti or naan bread.*
* **Refrigerate** *in an airtight container for up to 48 hours or freeze on day of cooking.*
* **Variations:** *Add 1 tablespoon of freshly chopped coriander in step 3.*

Coconut lentil dhal

This creamy dhal provides some iron and is a great dish that can be served early on or later in weaning and childhood as it purées and mashes well, or can be left as it is. As with the Lentil and spinach dhal (see above), the meal could be served with some well-diluted unsweetened orange juice to provide vitamin C to help the absorption of iron, as well as green vegetables.

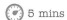 5 mins   25 mins   4–6 baby or 2 baby and 1 adult portion

ingredients

1 tbsp **vegetable oil**
60g (2oz) or 1 small **onion**, finely chopped
1 **garlic clove**, crushed (optional)
½ tsp **ground cumin**
100g (3½oz) split **red lentils**, rinsed
150ml (5fl oz) canned **coconut milk**
1 tbsp **tomato purée**

method

1 Heat the oil in a non-stick saucepan and fry the onion until soft. Add the garlic, if using.

2 Stir in the cumin and lentils and fry for 1 minute, stirring, before adding the coconut milk, 200ml (7fl oz) water, and tomato purée.

3 Bring to a simmer, stir, cover, and reduce the heat. Simmer for 15 minutes, and if it becomes a little dry, add 1–2 tablespoons of water.

4 Remove from the heat after 20 minutes, or when the lentils and onions are soft, and allow to cool a little.

5 Check the consistency and purée or mash, if needed. Serve your baby's portion, cooling, labelling, and freezing the remainder.

* **Serve** *with pieces of naan bread or chapatti, broccoli florets or green beans.*
* **Refrigerate** *in an airtight container for up to 24 hours or freeze.*
* **Variations:** *Stir in a ½ teaspoon of garam masala after 15 minutes of cooking.*

Creamy apricot dessert

Apricots provide vitamin A. In summer, use fresh ones to make this easy dessert. Out of season, use canned fruit in juice, draining off the juice before blending.

 2 mins   6 mins   1–2 baby portions and 1 adult

ingredients

250g (9oz) fresh **apricots**
75g (2½oz) **mascarpone cheese**

method

1 Wash the apricots, remove the stones, and quarter.

2 Place in a small saucepan with 2 tablespoons of water, adding another tablespoon if needed. Bring to a simmer, cover, stir, and cook for 4–5 minutes, or until tender.

3 Cool and blend until smooth. When the mixture has cooled, add the mascarpone and blend again. Spoon into little dishes and refrigerate.

✳ **Serve** *with pieces of fresh fruit.*

✳ **Refrigerate** *in an airtight container for up to 24 hours.*

✳ **Variations:** *Use fresh nectarines or peaches instead.*

Apply plums

In late summer, when plums are abundant, stew and freeze a few batches to use later in the year as desserts, breakfasts or to add to crumbles or pies. Depending on the type of plums you use, you may not need much juice for cooking.

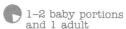 5 mins   2 baby and 2 adult portions

10–15 mins

ingredients

6 ripe **plums**
150ml (5fl oz) **cloudy apple juice**

method

1 Wash and halve the plums. Remove the stones and cut in half again.

2 Place in a small saucepan with the apple juice, cover, and simmer gently until soft. Cool and process lightly, if required, before serving.

✳ **Serve** *with 1 spoon of yogurt or fromage frais.*

✳ **Refrigerate** *in an airtight container for up to 48 hours or freeze on day of cooking when cool.*

Stewed apple and cranberries

Cranberries are a great source of protective plant substances, phenols. As they are sour, sweetened cranberries are used here with apples.

 10–12 mins   10–12 mins   3–4 baby portions

ingredients

1 medium **eating apple,** peeled, cored, and chopped into small pieces

25g (scant 1oz) **sweetened cranberries**

method

1 Place the apple pieces in a small saucepan along with the cranberries and 4 tablespoons of water. Cook over a low heat, stirring occasionally until softened.

2 Remove from the heat and cool. Mash or process to a suitable texture and serve.

✳ **Serve** *with yogurt, fromage frais or custard.*

✳ **Refrigerate** *in an airtight container for up to 48 hours or freeze on the day of cooking when cool.*

✳ **Variations:** *Use raisins instead of cranberries. Use the basis of this method to stew other fruits.*

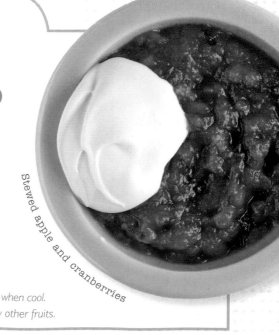

Stewed apple and cranberries

Fruity finger foods

As your baby grows more confident at grasping objects, you can give her a whole range of fruit to enjoy. Soft fruit is a great first finger food as it is naturally sweet so enjoyed by babies, and can be easily gnawed and chewed. Always stay with your baby when she is eating, especially if she is having finger foods, which she has a greater risk of choking on.

Apples and pears

Choose ripe and soft varieties, rather than firm ones.

Wash the fruits and peel with a vegetable peeler.

Quarter the fruits and remove the cores and any seeds. Slice into pieces your baby can easily hold.

Citrus fruit (oranges, clementines, and satsumas)

Given as whole segments, these can be difficult for a baby to eat because they are juicy and the membranes can cause choking. Prepare these fruits with care.

Remove all the peels and piths. Split the fruits into segments and remove the membranes surrounding each segment, checking for any pips.

Blueberries

Wash the berries and dry on kitchen paper. Cut in half.

Strawberries

Wash the fruits and remove the stalks. Cut in half, or slice if large.

Grapes

Choose the seedless variety, and wash thoroughly. Cut in half, pulling away the skin only if it is tough.

Kiwi fruit

Peel the fruit and cut in half lengthwise, removing the white core. Slice into pieces your baby can easily hold.

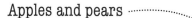

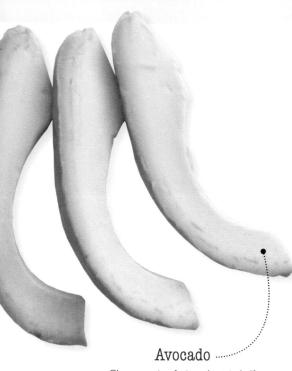

Stone fruit
(peaches, plums, apricots, and nectarines)

Choose ripe and tender fruits. Wash the fruits and peel off the skins, or drop the whole fruits in boiling water for 20 seconds first, and then peel.

Halve, remove the stones, and slice into pieces your baby can easily hold.

Avocado

Choose a ripe fruit and cut in half.

Remove the stone, cut in half lengthwise, and peel away the skin. Slice into pieces your baby can easily hold.

Papaya

Choose a small ripe papaya and cut in half.

Scoop out the seeds with a spoon and peel with a sharp knife or peeler.

Slice into pieces your baby can easily hold.

Mango

Choose a ripe mango. Cut away a "cheek" of the mango with a sharp knife, then slice the flesh into a crisscross pattern, cutting down to the peel, but not piercing it.

Push the peel inside out, and cut away the cubes with a knife.

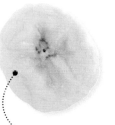
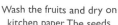

Bananas

Peel the banana and either cut into a few slices across the banana, or make batons by cutting down the length of the banana, then cutting again into 3–4cm (1–1½in) batons.

Raspberries

Wash the fruits and dry on kitchen paper. The seeds are tiny and can be eaten by your baby.

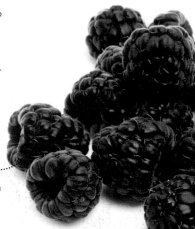

Mango lollies

Mango purée can be quickly frozen to make little lollies that are perfect for sitting outside on a warm day to eat. Rather than traditional lolly moulds, which are rather large, use egg cups, or very small pots, and pop in a wooden stick. Be prepared for a mess when your baby eats these: a bib is a must!

 5 mins   6–8 baby lollies ❄

ingredients

200g (7oz) **mango purée**,
  home-made (see p59)
  or shop-bought
juice of half a **lemon**

method

1 Mix the purée with the lemon juice and pour into 6–8 egg cups or moulds. Pop a wooden stick into the centre of each and freeze.

2 When frozen, place all the moulds in a container or bag to prevent frosting.

3 To serve, remove from the freezer and wait for a minute or so. To check if the lolly is ready for your baby, touch with your clean finger and make sure it does not stick.

✳ Variations: *Try different fruit purées such as apricot (see p60) or peach (see p61), or mix these with the mango.*

✳ Take care: Frozen foods such as lollies can stick to your child's lips if too cold. Remove from the freezer and allow to warm up a little, checking the lolly yourself before giving it to your baby.

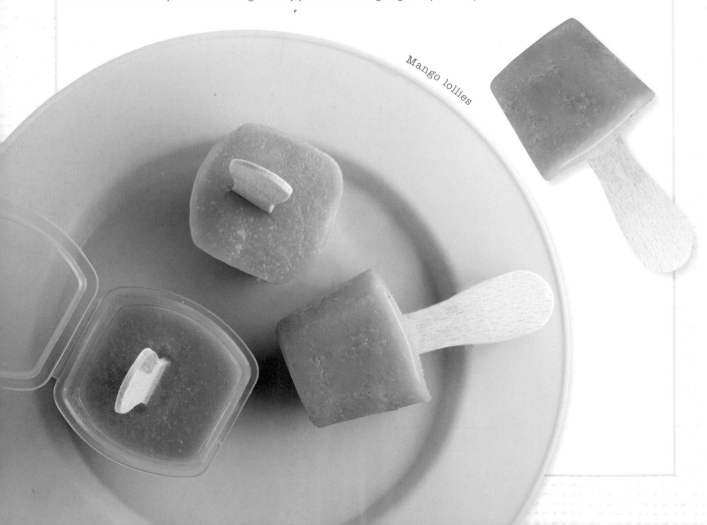

Mango lollies

Fruits of the forest iced yogurt

A bag of frozen fruits of the forest contains a range of berries and cherries high in protective polyphenols. For a younger baby, sieve out the seeds; for older babies and children, leave the seeds in as they provide fibre.

 5 mins 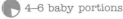 4–6 baby portions

ingredients

100g (3½oz) frozen **fruits of the forest**, defrosted

2 tsp **icing sugar**, if needed
100g (3½oz) full-fat, strained **Greek yogurt**

method

1 Purée the fruits until smooth and then pass through a sieve to remove the seeds. If very bitter, stir in 2 teaspoons of icing sugar.

2 Stir into the yogurt and pour into a plastic container suitable for the freezer. Cover and freeze until solid.

3 Remove from the freezer and place in the refrigerator for 10 minutes before serving to make the dessert easier to scoop.

✱ **Serve** with pieces of fruit or a plain sweet biscuit.
✱ The dessert can be frozen for up to 3 months.

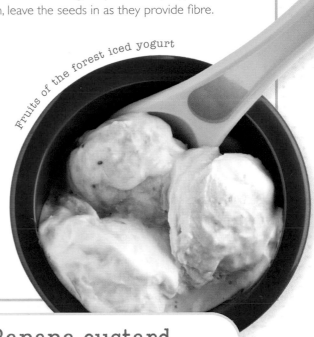

Fruits of the forest iced yogurt

Fruit fool

This uses cornflour custard instead of the traditional cream. It will work with many different seasonal fruits.

 5 mins 5 mins 2 baby and 1 adult portion

ingredients

10g (¼oz) **cornflour**
10g (¼oz) **sugar**
100ml (3½fl oz) **whole milk**
2 drops **vanilla extract**
125g (4½oz) **stewed fruit**, such as

rhubarb, stone fruit, or berries, sweetened if necessary
100g (3½oz) thick **plain yogurt** or **Greek yogurt**

method

1 Place the cornflour and sugar in a saucepan and stir in the milk. Heat gently, stirring continuously until you have a thick sauce. Remove from the heat and stir in the vanilla.

2 Blend the fruits to make a thick purée and stir into the cooled sauce. Gently mix in the yogurt and pour into little bowls. Cover and chill until required.

✱ **Serve** with pieces of fruit or a plain sweet biscuit.
✱ **Refrigerate** for up to 48 hours.

Banana custard

A simple milky dessert most babies (and some adults!) love. Milk contains lactose, a natural sugar, and bananas are also sweet, so although you may be tempted to add sugar, there is no need.

 2 mins 5 mins 2 baby portions

ingredients

1 dessertspoon **custard powder**

150 ml (5fl oz) **whole milk**
½ **banana**, sliced

method

1 Mix the custard powder with 2–3 tbsp of the milk in a large bowl.

2 Heat the remaining milk until almost boiling, then pour over the custard mixture, stirring all the time.

3 Return to the saucepan and heat, stirring all the time until thickened.

4 Divide the banana slices into 2 small bowls and pour the custard over the top. Allow to cool.

5 Keep in the fridge for up to 24 hours, bringing the dessert out of the fridge to warm a little before serving.

✱ **Refrigerate**, covered, for up to 24 hours.

Semolina pudding

Semolina pudding is a simple milky dessert that your baby will be able to eat easily. You can add stewed or puréed fruit to it, or serve it plain.

 2 mins 15 mins ◐ 2-3 baby portions

ingredients

10g (¼oz) **semolina**
150ml (5fl oz) **whole milk**

1 tsp **sugar**
few drops **vanilla extract**

method

1 Place all the ingredients except the vanilla extract in a small saucepan, and heat, stirring continuously, until thickened and the grains of semolina are soft.

2 Add the vanilla extract and cool slightly. Remove your baby's portion and serve warm.

✱ **Serve** *with apricot or fruit purée (see pp59–62).*
✱ **Refrigerate** *in a small airtight container for up to 24 hours.*

Ground rice pudding

This is made by mixing milk, ground rice, and a tiny quantity of sugar: an easy dessert that increases your baby's intake of calcium-rich milk. It's best made fresh, but extra can be refrigerated and microwave heated the next day, ensuring it's well stirred, then cooled.

 2 mins 10 mins 2-3 baby portions

ingredients

15g (½oz) **ground rice**
150ml (5fl oz) **whole milk**

1 tsp **sugar**
few drops **vanilla extract**

method

1 Place all the ingredients except the vanilla extract in a small saucepan. Heat, stirring continuously, until the mixture thickens and the rice is soft.

2 Add the vanilla extract and cool slightly. Remove your baby's portion and serve warm.

✱ **Serve** *with fruit purée (see pp59–62) or mashed fruits.*

Lemony ricotta pudding

Using only three ingredients, this dessert will be enjoyed by babies and parents alike. Think cheesecake, but healthier and simpler!

 5 mins   2 baby portions

ingredients

70g (2½oz) mild **ricotta cheese**
2 tsp **lemon curd**
1 **digestive biscuit**, crushed

method

1 Mix the ricotta with the lemon curd and stir in the biscuit crumbs.

2 Allow to stand for a few minutes to soften the crumbs a little, then serve or chill.

✱ **Serve** *with fresh fruit such as strawberries, peaches or pear.*
✱ **Refrigerate** *in an airtight container for up to 24 hours.*

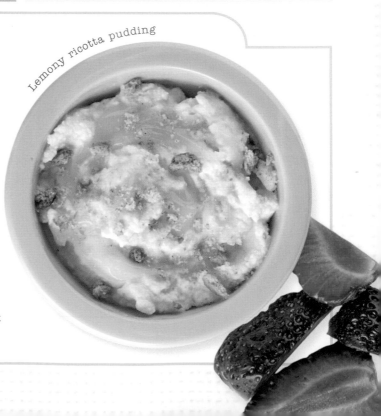
Lemony ricotta pudding

Rice pudding

A traditional nursery favourite, rice pudding is a calcium-rich, easily digested dessert.

 5 mins   2 hours   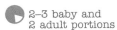 2–3 baby and 2 adult portions

ingredients

25g (scant 1oz) **butter**
25g (scant 1oz) **sugar**
50g (1¾oz) **short-grain rice**

500ml (16fl oz) **whole milk**
2 strips **lemon peel**
1 **bay leaf**
grated **nutmeg**

method

1 Preheat the oven to 140°C (275°F/Gas 1). Butter a 1 litre (1¾ pints) ovenproof dish.

2 Place all the ingredients except the nutmeg in a saucepan and slowly bring to a simmer, stirring often. Reduce the heat and simmer for 5 minutes. Stir, pour into the greased dish, and place in the oven.

3 After 30 minutes, remove, stir, and return to the oven. Repeat after another 30 minutes, but remove the bay leaf and lemon peel, and top with the grated nutmeg.

4 Return to the oven for 30–45 minutes, or until the pudding is set but slightly wobbly. Cool before serving.

✱ **Serve** *with a spoon of stewed apricots or plums (see p129).*
✱ **Refrigerate** *for up to 48 hours. Not suitable for freezing.*
✱ **Variation:** *Add 2 tablespoons of raisins.*

Fruit with chocolate dipping sauce

This is a cornflour-thickened chocolaty milk sauce in which your baby will enjoy dunking fingers of fruit, or just fingers!

 5 mins   5 mins   2–3 baby portions

ingredients

1 tbsp **cornflour**
1 rounded tbsp **drinking chocolate powder**, or 1 level tbsp **cocoa powder** and 2 tsp **sugar**

150ml (5fl oz) **whole milk**
2–3 drops **vanilla extract**
assorted fruits such as **mango**, **strawberry**, and **grapes**, sliced

method

1 Place the cornflour and chocolate powder in a small saucepan and slowly stir in the milk.

2 Add the vanilla extract then heat, stirring continuously, until the sauce thickens.

3 Pour into 2–3 small bowls, allow to cool, and serve with fruit pieces for dipping.

✱ **Refrigerate** *the chocolate custard for 48 hours, but cut up the fruits just before serving.*

Chocolate rice pudding

Worth the wait, this chocolate-rich rice pudding provides essential calcium, and you and your baby will enjoy its creamy flavour.

 5 mins   2 hours   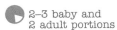 2–3 baby and 2 adult portions

ingredients

25g (scant 1oz) **butter**
25g (scant 1oz) **sugar**
50g (1¾oz) **short-grain rice**
500ml (16fl oz) **whole milk**
10g (¼oz) **cocoa powder**

method

1 Preheat the oven to 140°C (275°F/Gas 1). Butter a 1 litre (1¾ pints) ovenproof dish.

2 Place all the ingredients in a saucepan and slowly bring to simmering point, stirring frequently, making sure the cocoa is well absorbed. Reduce the heat and simmer for 5 minutes.

3 Stir well then pour into the greased dish, and place in the oven. After 30 minutes, remove, stir, and return to the oven. Repeat after another 30 minutes.

4 Return to the oven for another 30–45 minutes, or until the pudding is just set but slightly wobbly. Allow the pudidng to cool a little before serving.

✱ **Serve** *with a few slices of banana.*
✱ **Variation:** *Add 2 tablespoons of raisins.*

Introducing *Stage 3*

By the third stage of weaning, which is usually around nine to 12 months, your baby will be used to having regular meals and be fitting into some family mealtimes. Eating together has many positive benefits for him. Remember, though, that you need to model your behaviour for your baby, as he will pick up on your table manners, whether good or bad!

Progressing through the third stage

In this third stage, the texture of your baby's food changes from being mashed with a few soft lumps and sometimes minced to being minced more of the time or simply chopped. He will also be gaining more confidence drinking from a cup. Keep offering foods that have been tricky to introduce previously rather than write them off. Research shows that the more times your baby is exposed to a food, the more likely he is to eat it.

What your baby needs now

- Milk is still the mainstay of his diet; he needs a minimum of 500ml (17fl oz) each day, or 2–3 breastfeeds.

- Your baby's appetite has grown to meet his energy needs as he becomes more mobile. Make sure that energy-rich foods such as full-fat cheese and dairy products feature in his daily diet.

- He should have a wide range of vegetables and continue to eat plenty of fruit.

- Your baby should be able to eat a good range of finger foods now, and you can offer some harder textures, including raw vegetables.

- As your baby approaches one year, there will be more family foods that he will be able to eat. At this point, it's important to remember not to add salt or salted stocks to foods he'll be eating with you. You can remove his portion before adding seasoning for the rest of the family, or add salt at the table for yourself if you need it. As well as being unhealthy for your baby, bear in mind too that although a dish may taste bland or in need of seasoning to you, it won't to him as he doesn't have your experience of taste.

Your independent feeder

As your baby approaches his first birthday, he will have made an amazing amount of progress in many areas of development, and these changes will help him develop the ability to feed himself.

From around eight months, he will also be learning to curl his lip round a beaker or cup, and as his coordination improves he will be able to drink water from a cup without a lid at his high chair without too many spills.

His pincer grip, which develops around nine months, will be getting stronger so he is able to pick up finger foods with his finger and thumb rather than his fist. This also means that he will be able to pick up smaller finger foods such as raisins more easily. As his coordination improves he'll be able to use a spoon to convey food to his mouth, but this takes some practice.

Your baby will be better at chewing, and should be able to cope with lumps in food as well as breaking off chunks of finger food and moving them around his mouth to chew.

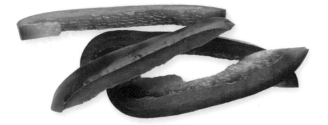

STAGE 3 – at a glance

TEXTURE	During the third stage of weaning, the texture of your baby's food changes from being **mashed** with **some soft lumps** and **occasionally minced** to being **minced** more of the time or **chopped**.
INTRODUCE	Introduce more flavours into his food, giving him more mild spices and adding herbs so he gets used to stronger tastes.
AVOID	Do not give processed meats such as sausages and ham, honey, liver, and whole nuts (see p19).

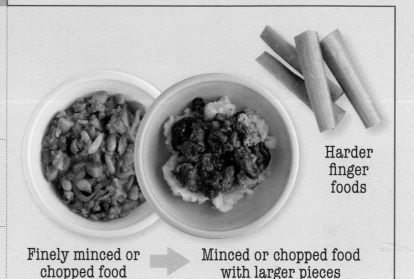

Finely minced or chopped food → Minced or chopped food with larger pieces

Harder finger foods

Portions for older babies

As your baby's diet becomes more varied and complex, he will eat more finger foods and meals composed of many food groups. The portions guide table for this stage is therefore based on the four main food groups (see p13). Babies, like everyone else, have individual appetites, so the table is just a guide to what the range of intakes may be for this age group.

FOOD GROUP	WHICH MEAL?	TYPICAL AMOUNT FOR 10–12 MONTH OLD
Vegetables	Eat at lunch and dinner	1–2 tbsp or as finger food
Fruits	Any, but at least 2 meals a day	1–2 tbsp or as finger food
Grains, cereals, potatoes, and pasta	Eat some at every meal	2–4 tbsp per meal
Meat, poultry, fish, eggs, and pulses	Eat at 2 meals a day	1–2 tbsp for meat, fish and poultry, per meal 2–3 tbsp if pulses or nuts, per meal
Milk	Throughout day	500ml (17fl oz) formula milk or 2–3 breastfeeds
Dairy – yogurt, fromage frais, and milk desserts	Once or twice a day as dessert or breakfast	2–4 tbsp dairy foods
Finger foods	With meals or occasional snack	Half to one slice bread 1–2 baby rice cakes 2 strawberries, 5 halved grapes, 1 sliced plum Quarter pear or apple 2–3 small vegetable batons
High-fat and high-sugar foods	Not suitable	Not suitable

Common-sense feeding

In recent years, much research has been carried out to see if there is a link between the growth in childhood obesity and the way in which parents approach feeding babies and toddlers. Various studies have come up with theories, but results are conflicting with no conclusive large-scale study. What is clear is that families have individual approaches and attitudes to food, some preferring the routine of set mealtimes from the outset, while others are more relaxed. Your job as a parent is to find an approach that works for you while ensuring that your baby is confident trying new foods that lead him to enjoy a balanced, healthy diet.

What type of parent are you?

Studies have shown that early childhood preferences help determine food preferences for life. While this is useful information, it also puts a certain amount of pressure on parents. Armed with the knowledge that if their baby eats broccoli at seven months he is more likely to eat it at seven years, many parents feel a big responsibility to get feeding right, perhaps encouraging them to put pressure on their babies during mealtimes that could be counterproductive.

Research has tried to identify whether parents who are more relaxed about weaning bring up babies who are more confident about trying new foods. Or alternatively whether parents who adopt adult healthy eating guidelines themselves mistakenly restrict the food intake of their children. They may cut out certain nutrients, such as fats, that their baby needs to grow and develop healthily.

Whatever your approach to food, being aware of how your baby develops tastes and preferences (see pp48–9) and learns to eat a varied and healthy diet should help you to work out a feeding regime that works for you both. So if you're a parent who likes order, the mess involved in weaning may be challenging. However, recognizing that making a mess is a natural stage in your baby's development that helps him practise his coordination and eventually leads to successful self-feeding can help curb your desire to mop up constantly. Putting paper or a splash mat on the floor and a bib on your baby gives you some control over mess while your baby has the freedom to explore his food.

Getting it right

Often, anxiety about making sure their baby eats well causes parents to forget common-sense advice:

- Try to be relaxed. If you are stressed about mealtimes, your baby will pick this up. Remind yourself that babies can take several tries before accepting a food, so don't be disheartened if food is rejected. Make eating a social event: talk to your baby, smile, and ensure that mealtimes have positive associations.

- Don't pressurize your baby to eat; he'll show you when he is hungry and respond by eating. Swooping spoons and over-persuasion may inadvertently decrease his motivation to eat.

- Banning foods can make them more desirable. Parents who restrict foods can find that when their child is older and goes to other homes, he over-indulges on foods off limits at home. You don't want your child to have biscuits each day, but an occasional treat for toddlers is fine.

- Don't expect your baby to eat foods you don't eat. If you never eat your greens, he won't either. Do you need to look at your diet, too?

- Let your baby have some control: the more you restrict or control his food the more likely he is to develop emotional eating behaviours.

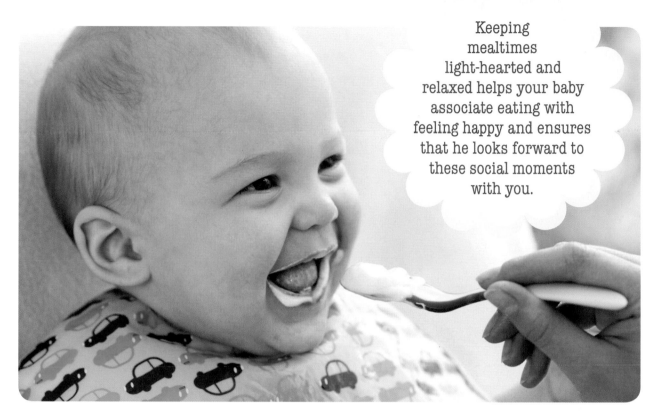

Keeping mealtimes light-hearted and relaxed helps your baby associate eating with feeling happy and ensures that he looks forward to these social moments with you.

Your baby's temperament

Child psychologists and nutritionists have been looking at whether babies' temperaments have an impact on the way they receive food or are fed, and whether this influences whether they are more likely to become overweight in later childhood.

Some of the types of questions researchers have investigated are:

• Do babies who are difficult to settle become overweight as older children because milk or food is used to comfort them?

• Do some babies respond to parents' over-persuasive attempts to feed them by screaming during feeding or holding food in their mouths, and could this resistance affect growth?

• Are smiley, sociable babies easier to feed because their parents are more relaxed about feeding, or are they more relaxed themselves and this makes weaning easier for their parents?

Different studies have shown a range of answers, but one large study in the UK, called the Gateshead Millenium study, which followed babies from birth up to seven to eight years, showed that there was no evidence that a baby's temperament was likely to lead to him being a greater weight in later childhood. Parents can therefore be reassured that their baby's temperament will not be a barrier to achieving a healthy, varied diet, and that setting up good habits is valuable as these can last into the adult years.

Eating *together*

The phrase "family mealtime" may conjure up a picture of a harmonious family sitting round a table eating healthy food, smiling, and enjoying each other's company. Or it may not! Whether your own childhood experience of mealtimes was a positive or negative one, it is known that children who take part in family meals benefit in a number of ways. It doesn't matter if the meal is a bit chaotic, and manners aren't perfect – it just matters that the family are trying to be together in a shared act.

Why family meals matter

Many studies have looked at whether eating together as a family makes a difference to family life, and evidence suggests that children who take part in family meals benefit in several ways. When babies and toddlers eat with the family, they are less likely to be overweight and more likely to eat a healthier diet. This is because family meals are more likely to be nutritionally balanced.

There are also social and psychological benefits. Children who eat meals with the family appear to have improved psychological wellbeing and more positive family interactions. This underpins the fact that mealtimes are not just eating occasions, but social events, too. When family life is busy and hectic, having set times when you eat together provides an opportunity for you to catch up as a family, and establishing family meals early on will benefit your child over the years.

Eating together as a family may also help you to adopt a healthier diet. If you're used to eating regular ready meals or processed meats, you may have to review your eating habits when your baby joins you at the table. Like it or not, your baby mimics what you do and say, so you can use this opportunity to show him that you eat a wide variety of different healthy meals.

Let your baby watch you prepare his meal and tell him what you are doing to engage his imagination. This way, he'll learn to relate the food in its raw state to the meal that he eats.

Setting an example

Now may be a good time to examine your own feelings about food. If you are a restrictive eater yourself, perhaps you have certain food issues or are dieting, take care not to talk about foods being "good" or "bad". Your baby needs to eat a healthy diet that includes energy-dense foods. This may include foods you're avoiding while dieting, such as cheese, oils or fats, but it's important for him to have some of these in his daily diet.

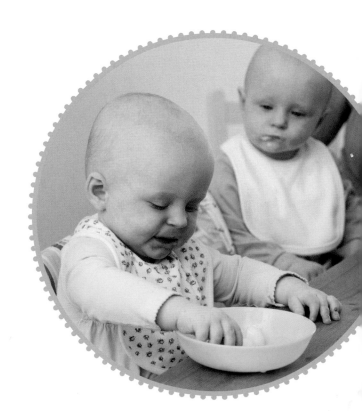

Making it work

While eating together is the ideal, busy modern lives mean this is often impractical. If you and/or your partner work late, eating together as a family during the week may not always work for you. Rather than feel guilty, think about ways to build in some dedicated family eating occasions:

- Sit down at the table for a meal every Saturday or Sunday, inviting others to join you occasionally. Your baby benefits from these social occasions as he listens to conversation and watches behaviour, observing table manners as well as learning language skills.

- Eat lunch with your baby. Rather than tidy up the kitchen while your baby is having lunch, make time to have a sandwich, too. Let him try yours if he wants to.

- If you are cooking for the rest of the family, select some suitable finger foods for your baby to have at the same time as your meal, or adapt the meal so he can have the same. This is often just a case of leaving out the salt, or removing a portion for your baby before adding salt, and chopping or mashing the food. This leads the way to your baby joining in with family mealtimes by one year of age.

- Invite older children to eat at the table; whether these are your own, cousins or friends, babies love to be with other children, and this makes a simple mealtime into a hugely enjoyable occasion for him. He may want to eat what they are eating, so you might need to adjust the menu. Toddlers can also benefit from being with children who have left the picky stage behind.

- Make food and the family the focus: turn off the television or computer while you eat so your baby isn't distracted.

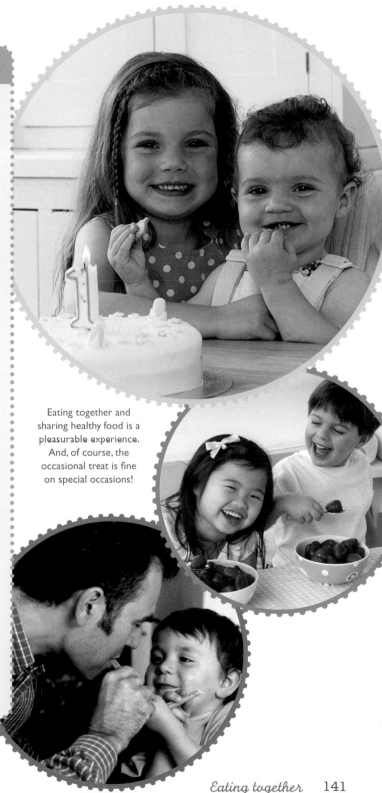

Eating together and sharing healthy food is a pleasurable experience. And, of course, the occasional treat is fine on special occasions!

day-by-day meal planner
Week 1

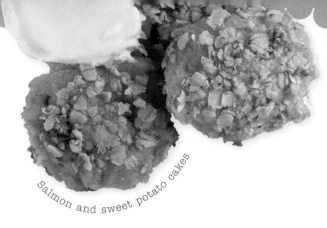

Salmon and sweet potato cakes

Monday

Breakfast
Scrambled egg p99 and toast with melon pieces

Lunch
Baked potato with salmon, yogurt, and cucumber p176 and steamed green beans
Semolina pudding p134 with mashed kiwi fruit

Dinner
Beef with prunes p116 with mashed potato and steamed broccoli
Exotic fruit salad p191

Tuesday

Breakfast
Vanilla and banana smoothie p171 with satsuma pieces

Lunch
Pea and mint soup p181 with cheese scone p104
Fruit fool p133

Dinner
Cowboy beans with cornmeal topping p188 and steamed green beans
Blackberry apple cobbler p195

Wednesday

Breakfast
Simple muesli p169 with milk and banana slices

Lunch
Butternut or pumpkin and tomato soup p180 with egg and cress sandwich p175
Fromage frais with berries

Dinner
Shepherd's pie p185 with roast carrot and pepper fingers
Baked spiced peaches p190

Thursday

Breakfast
Puffed rice cereal with raisins and milk with mango pieces p131

Lunch
Ham and pineapple pizza p179 with halved cherry tomatoes
Chocolate rice pudding p135

Dinner
Salmon and sweet potato cakes p121 with tzatkiki dip and cucumber sticks
Stewed plums p129

Friday

Breakfast
Date porridge p98
with orange segments

Lunch
Beef meatballs in tomato sauce p185
with pasta shapes and steamed cauliflower
Mandarin jelly p192

Dinner
Bulghur wheat with lamb and aubergine
p184 with cucumber sticks
Yogurt and mashed berries

Saturday

Breakfast
Fruits of the forest smoothie p168
Toast and cream cheese p100

Lunch
Crispy salmon fingers p186 with mashed
potato and peas
Crushed canned pineapple with yogurt

Dinner
Butternut squash risotto p122 with
steamed courgette fingers
Fromage frais and fruit purée pp59–62

Sunday

Breakfast
Savoury muffin p170
with slices of soft pear p130

Lunch
Macaroni cheese p125
with halved cherry tomatoes
Mandarins with rice pudding p135

Dinner
Beef meatballs in tomato sauce p185
with pasta shapes and steamed broccoli
Stewed apple and raisins p129

Offer your
baby a drink with his
meals – either his usual milk
or water in a lidded cup. If you
wish to give juice, give
unsweetened fruit juice diluted
one part juice to 10 parts
water.

Other ideas this week Oat porridge p98 with banana slices • Toast and peanut butter p101 • Baked beans on toast p173 • Ricotta, tomato, and basil sandwich p174 with carrot sticks • Chicken and pasta with creamy sauce p183 • Chicken Provençale p112 • Baked egg custard p195

day-by-day meal planner

Week 2

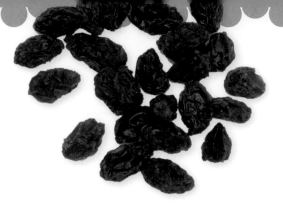

Monday

Breakfast
Bircher muesli p98
with banana slices

Lunch
Carrot and coriander soup p181 with
ricotta, tomato, and basil sandwich p174
Yogurt with fruit purée pp59–62

Dinner
Vegetarian shepherd's pie p189
with steamed broccoli
Baked egg custard p195

Tuesday

Breakfast
Banana bread p168 and cream cheese
with clementine segments

Lunch
Sardines on toast p173 with
cucumber fingers
Apply plums p129

Dinner
Herby lamb with vegetables p114
with soft potato and parsnips
Fromage frais with
apricot purée p60

Wednesday

Breakfast
Apricot porridge p68
with soft ready-to-eat apricot pieces

Lunch
Cauliflower cheese p125
with bread and butter
Stewed summer berries p191

Dinner
Fruity chicken p112 with potato pieces
and steamed green beans
Apple sponge pudding p193

Thursday

Breakfast
Mixed spice drop scone with butter
p99 with soft pear pieces p130

Lunch
Pancake p192 with Mexican beans p177
with steamed carrot fingers
Yogurt with mashed blueberries

Dinner
Salmon and dill risotto p186
with avocado fingers p131
Mandarin lolly p132

Friday

Breakfast
Baked egg with cheese and tomato p172
wlth clementine pieces

Lunch
Tuna and avocado sandwich p175
with halved cherry tomatoes
Fromage frais with fruit purée pp59–62

Dinner
Chicken mini-burgers p183 with peach chutney
p182 and cucumber and pepper fingers
Baked stuffed apple p190

Saturday

Breakfast
Wheat biscuit with milk p70 and mashed banana
with papaya or melon pieces

Lunch
Cottage cheese dip p107
with steamed salmon flakes p106 and bread
Stewed apple and raisins p129

Dinner
Bulghur wheat with lamb and aubergine p184
with steamed broccoli florets
Yogurt with fruit purée pp59–62

Sunday

Breakfast
Baby blueberry pancakes p169
with banana slices

Lunch
Cheese and tomato tortilla/wrap p177
with cucumber fingers
Mandarins with rice pudding p135

Dinner
Normandy pork p113 with potato pieces
and steamed green beans
Stewed apple and raisins p129
with custard

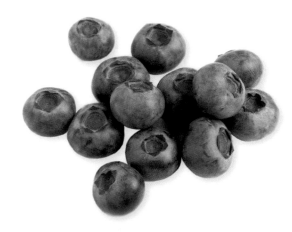

Other ideas this week Mango smoothie p171 with toast • Baby falafel p110 with home-made hummus p111 •
Leek and potato soup p180 with bread fingers • Creamy avocado pasta p188 with broccoli
• Greek baked fish p120 with cooked spinach and potatoes • Apple and pear slices p130

day-by-day meal planner

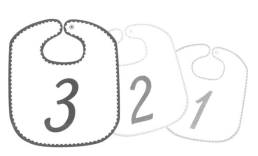

Week **3** 2 1

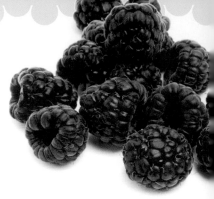

Monday

Breakfast
Raspberry porridge p99
with raspberries

Lunch
Creamy avocado pasta p188
with halved cherry tomatoes
Yogurt with strawberry slices

Dinner
Simple fish pie p187 with
steamed courgettes
Pear and raisin oat crumble p193
and custard

Tuesday

Breakfast
Carrot muffin p171
with halved grapes

Lunch
Pea and mint soup p181 with
ricotta, tomato, and basil sandwich p174
Pear or peach slices pp130–31

Dinner
Lentil and spinach dhal p128 with rice
and steamed carrots
Fromage frais with
mashed berries

Wednesday

Breakfast
Puffed rice cereal with milk
and sliced banana

Lunch
Pesto, tomato, and mozzarella pizza p178
with cucumber and red pepper fingers
Stewed summer berries p191 with
ice cream

Dinner
Herby lamb with vegetables p114
with steamed sweet potato fingers
Pear and raisin oat crumble p193
and custard

Thursday

Breakfast
Scrambled egg p99 and buttered toast
with clementine segments

Lunch
Home-made hummus p111 with pitta
bread and red pepper fingers
Yogurt with pitted prunes on side

Dinner
Chicken and pasta with creamy sauce p183
with steamed broccoli and carrots
Ground rice pudding p134
and fruit purée pp59–62

Friday

Breakfast
Mango smoothie p171 with toast
and cream cheese p100

Lunch
Simple fish pie p187 with
steamed broccoli and carrots
Melon pieces

Dinner
Pork with pineapple p114 with
rice and steamed broccoli
Apricot and almond
pudding p194

Saturday

Breakfast
Spicy banana toast p100
with apple slices

Lunch
Mackerel and tomato pizza p179
with carrot and red pepper fingers
Stewed summer berries p191

Dinner
Shepherd's pie with beef p185
with steamed cauliflower florets
Baked spiced peach p190

Sunday

Breakfast
Sweetcorn and tomato fritter p172
with fruits of the forest smoothie p168

Lunch
Pineapple and cheese on toast p173
with cucumber and halved cherry tomatoes
Pear or plum slices pp130–31

Dinner
Crispy salmon fingers p186 with mashed
potato, cucumber, and avocado dip p105
Passion fruit and mango dessert p191

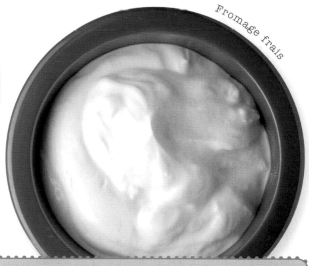

Fromage frais

Other ideas this week Wheat biscuit p70 with fruit • Tuna and avocado sandwich p175 with steamed courgettes • Fruity couscous with peanut sauce p189 • Bulghur wheat with currants and chickpeas p187• Beef ragu p115 with pasta and broccoli • Semolina p134 with fruit

day-by-day meal planner
Week 4 3 2 1

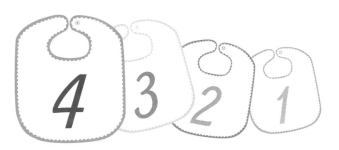

Monday

Breakfast
Banana bread p168 with cream cheese with papaya or soft pear slices pp130–31

Lunch
Pineapple and cheese on toast p173 with red pepper fingers
Stewed apple and cranberries p129

Dinner
Chicken Provençale p112 with soft cooked potato and courgette pieces
Baked egg custard p195 with berries

Tuesday

Breakfast
Baked egg with cheese and tomato p172 with halved grapes

Lunch
Baked beans on toast p173
Stewed summer berries p191

Dinner
Creamy vegetarian mince p126 with pasta shapes and steamed broccoli
Pear and raisin oat crumble p193

Wednesday

Breakfast
Fruits of the forest smoothie p168 with toast and cream cheese p100

Lunch
Cauliflower cheese p125 with bread and butter and halved cherry tomatoes
Melon or pear pieces p130

Dinner
Crispy salmon fingers p186 with home-made tomato salsa p182, mashed potatoes, and steamed green beans
Yogurt and kiwi slices

Thursday

Breakfast
Date porridge p98 with banana slices

Lunch
Turkey and red pepper patties p184 with home-made tomato salsa p182, bread and butter, and cucumber fingers
Semolina pudding p134 and mandarins

Dinner
Baby's first lamb tagine p115 with couscous p102, steamed carrots and broccoli
Passion fruit and mango dessert p191

Friday

Breakfast
Wheat biscuit with milk p70 and apricot purée p60
Kiwi slices

Lunch
Greek baked fish p120 with soft potato and broccoli pieces
Apple sponge pudding p193 with custard

Dinner
Creamy vegetable korma p126 with rice and strips of naan bread
Fruits of the forest iced yogurt p133

Saturday

Breakfast
Baked egg with cheese and tomato p172 with clementine segments

Lunch
Mushroom and onion pizza p178 with carrot and pepper sticks
Bread and butter pudding p194 with raisins

Dinner
Salmon and dill risotto p186 with steamed broccoli
Whole or mashed berries

Sunday

Breakfast
Simple muesli p169 with two soft ready-to-eat apricots

Lunch
Baked potatoes with spicy chicken and vegetables p176
with cucumber fingers
Banana custard p133

Dinner
Beef and onion casserole p116 with potatoes and broccoli
Stewed apple and cranberries p129 with custard

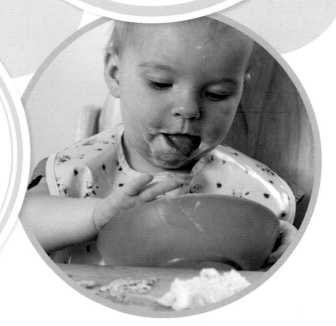

Other ideas this week Baby blueberry pancakes p169 • Pea and mint soup p181 with pitta • Hard-boiled egg with buttered toast p69 Garden vegetable risotto p127 • Beef meatballs in tomato sauce p185 with broccoli • Apricot and almond pudding p194

day-by-day meal planner
Week

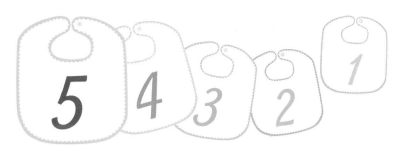

5 4 3 2 1

Monday

Breakfast
Simple muesli p169 with yogurt or milk and banana slices

Lunch
Carrot and coriander soup p181 with bread and butter fingers
Fromage frais with berries

Dinner
Pancakes p192 with salmon, yogurt, and cucumber p176 with steamed carrot fingers
Canned apricots and custard

Tuesday

Breakfast
Scrambled egg p99 with buttered toast p69 and kiwi slices

Lunch
Mackerel and tomato pizza p179 with avocado fingers
Yogurt with apple purée p59

Dinner
Bulghur wheat with currants and chickpeas p187 with steamed sugarsnaps
Apply plums p129 and yogurt

Wednesday

Breakfast
Baby blueberry pancakes p169 with blueberries

Lunch
Little sausage and apple balls p106 with home-made tomato salsa p182, bread and butter, and carrot fingers
Fruit fool p133

Dinner
Lentil and spinach dhal p128 with rice, chapatti fingers, and green beans
Mango or peach slices p131

Thursday

Breakfast
Banana bread p168 and cream cheese with soft pear pieces

Lunch
Pea and mint soup p181 with cheesy polenta twigs p108
Canned mandarins with yogurt

Dinner
Shepherd's pie (with lamb or beef) p185 with steamed swede fingers
Rice pudding p135 with mashed berries

Friday

Breakfast
Simple muesli p169 with yogurt or milk
and vanilla and banana smoothie p171

Lunch
Beef meatballs in tomato sauce p185
with pasta shapes and broccoli florets
Stewed summer berries p191 with custard

Dinner
Salmon and sweet potato cakes p121
with tzatziki, pasta shapes, and
steamed broccoli
Exotic fruit salad p191

Saturday

Breakfast
Puffed rice cereal and milk
with clementine segments

Lunch
Egg and cress sandwich p175
with soft ready-to-eat apricots
Lemony ricotta pudding p134

Dinner
Chicken and pasta with creamy sauce
p183 with steamed broccoli
Apple sponge pudding p193
and custard

Sunday

Breakfast
Baked egg with cheese and tomato p172
with bread and butter

Lunch
Baby falafel p110 with bread and butter,
avocado dip p105, and red pepper fingers
Creamy apricot dessert p129

Dinner
Chicken and broccoli p74 with rice
Fruit fool p133

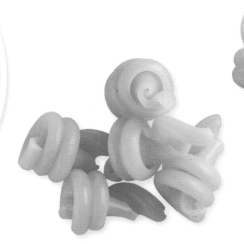

Other ideas this week Carrot muffin p171 with mango slices p131 • Mushroom and onion pizza p178 with carrot sticks • Baked potato with cheese and tomato p177 • Herby lamb with vegetables p114 Fruity couscous with peanut sauce p189 • Baked stuffed apple p190

day-by-day meal planner
Week 6

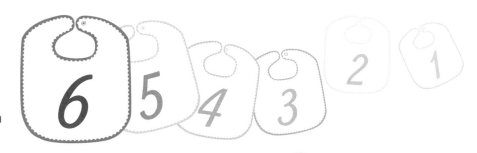

Monday

Breakfast
Baked egg with cheese and tomato
p172 with canned peach slices

Lunch
Sardines on toast p173
with red pepper/cucumber sticks
Fromage frais with stewed fruit p129

Dinner
Beef meatballs in tomato sauce p185
with pasta shapes and
steamed broccoli
Fruit and custard

Tuesday

Breakfast
Bircher muesli p98
with dried apple slices

Lunch
Macaroni cheese p125
with steamed broccoli/carrots
Apricot and almond pudding p194

Dinner
Salmon and dill risotto p186
with avocado fingers
Mango lolly p132

Wednesday

Breakfast
Spicy peach breakfast p96
with banana slices

Lunch
Cowboy beans with cornmeal topping
p188 with steamed carrots
Fromage frais with strawberry slices

Dinner
Normandy pork p113 with couscous p102,
steamed cauliflower, and green beans
Berries with chocolate dipping
sauce p135

Thursday

Breakfast
Baby blueberry pancakes p169 with cream cheese
Mango or peach pieces p131

Lunch
Baked potato with spicy chicken and vegetables
p176 with red pepper and cucumber fingers
Yogurt with mashed kiwi

Dinner
Sweet potatoes with sardines and peas p117
with steamed carrot and green beans
Stewed summer berries p191
or pear pieces p130

Friday

Breakfast
Wheat biscuit with milk p70 and raisins
with pear slices p130

Lunch
Coconut lentil dhal p128 with rice,
pitta bread, and green beans
Banana custard p133

Dinner
Fruity chicken p112 with mashed
sweetcorn, steamed sweet potato pieces,
and broccoli
Pear or apple pieces p130

Saturday

Breakfast
Scrambled egg p99 with buttered toast
with clementine segments

Lunch
Tuna and avocado sandwich p175
with cucumber fingers
Yogurt with sliced fruit

Dinner
Shepherd's pie (beef or lamb) p185
with steamed sugar snaps
Baked stuffed apple p190

Sunday

Breakfast
Mango smoothie p171
with carrot muffin p171

Lunch
Leek and potato soup p180
with cheese scone p104
Sliced banana or berries

Dinner
Greek baked fish p120 with mashed
potato, broccoli, and peas
Chocolate rice pudding p135

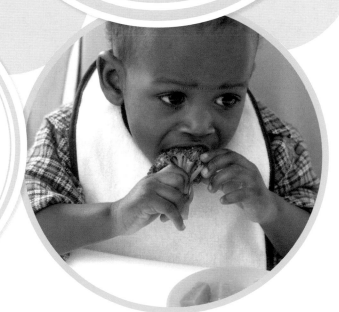

Other ideas this week Date porridge p98 with clementines • Carrot and coriander soup p181 with bread and butter • Fruity couscous with peanut sauce p189 • Vegetarian shepherd's pie p189 • Simple fish pie p187 with steamed green beans • Exotic fruit salad p191

day-by-day meal planner
Week 7 6 5

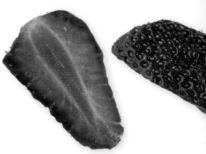
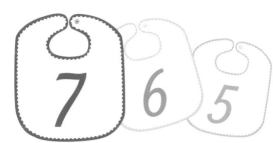

Monday

Breakfast
Raspberry porridge p99
with banana slices

Lunch
Cheesy tomato risotto p124
with pepper and carrot sticks
Creamy apricot dessert p129

Dinner
Simple fish pie p187
with steamed broccoli
Pear and raisin oat crumble
p193 with custard

Tuesday

Breakfast
Banana bread p168
with cream cheese and fruits of
the forest smoothie p168

Lunch
Baked potato or wrap with
Mexican beans p177 with cucumber
Fruit fool p133

Dinner
Beef meatballs in tomato sauce
p185 with pasta shapes and
steamed broccoli
Baked spiced peach p190
with yogurt

Wednesday

Breakfast
Buttered brioche slices with yogurt
and strawberry slices

Lunch
Italian tomato and tuna mash p120 with
cooked spinach
Orange segments with fromage frais

Dinner
Chicken mini-burgers with fruity sauce p183
with steamed broccoli
Stewed apple and cranberries p129
with custard

Thursday

Breakfast
Simple muesli p169 with milk or yogurt
with papaya or mango slices p131

Lunch
Creamy vegetarian mince p126 with
steamed sweet potato and green beans
Mandarin jelly p192

Dinner
Shepherd's pie p185
with steamed parsnip or swede
Fruits of the forest smoothie p168

Friday

Breakfast
Puffed rice cereal with milk
with soft ready-to-eat prunes

Lunch
Beef ragu p115 with pasta shapes and
steamed mangetout
Fruit fool p133

Dinner
Butternut squash risotto p122 with cooked
spinach and steamed courgette fingers
Blackberry apple cobbler p195
with yogurt

Saturday

Breakfast
Mixed spice drop scone p99 with
butter and strawberry slices

Lunch
Scrambled egg p99 on English muffin
with carrot or pepper sticks
Semolina pudding p134 with apricot
purée p60

Dinner
Pork with pineapple p114 and rice
with steamed celery and green beans
Fruits of the forest
iced yogurt p133

Sunday

Breakfast
Stewed apple and raisins p129 with toast
fingers and hard-boiled egg wedges p69

Lunch
Vegetarian shepherd's pie p189
with steamed cauliflower
Yogurt with raspberries

Dinner
Creamy salmon and pasta p121
with steamed sugar snaps
Pancakes p192 with stewed fruit p129

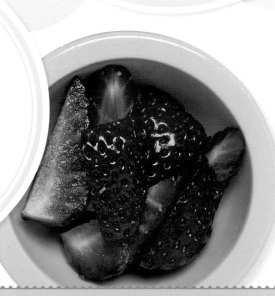
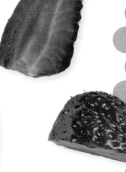

Other ideas this week — Baby blueberry pancakes p169 • Sweetcorn and tomato fritters p172 • Pea and mint soup p181 • Chicken and pasta with creamy sauce p183 with broccoli • Cowboy beans with cornmeal topping p188 • Stewed summer berries p191

day-by-day meal planner
Week 8 7 6 5

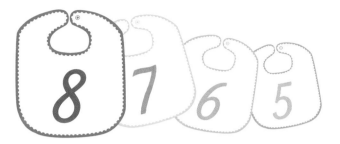
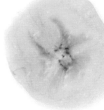

Monday

Breakfast
Toast and cream cheese p100
with orange segments

Lunch
Ham and pineapple pizza p179 with
pepper sticks
Stewed summer berries p191 and yogurt

Dinner
Creamy vegetable korma p126
with strips of naan bread
Rice pudding p135 with dried fruit

Tuesday

Breakfast
Simple muesli p169
with banana slices

Lunch
Salmon and sweet potato cakes p121
with tzatziki and cucumber sticks
Banana custard p133

Dinner
Chicken and pasta with creamy sauce
p183 with broccoli
Rice pudding p135 with
canned mandarins

Wednesday

Breakfast
Wheat biscuit with milk p70
with soft dried apple pieces

Lunch
Bulghur wheat with currants and chickpeas
p187 with tomato quarters
Banana with chocolate dipping sauce p135

Dinner
Beef ragu p115 with pasta shapes and
mashed peas
Passion fruit and
mango dessert p191

Thursday

Breakfast
Toast with hrad-boiled egg wedges p69
and kiwi slices

Lunch
Creamy salmon and pasta p121
with steamed green beans
Yogurt with stewed summer stone fruit
p129

Dinner
Herby lamb with vegetables p114
with steamed potato pieces
Bread and butter pudding p194

Friday

Breakfast
Yogurt with mashed berries
with bread and butter fingers

Lunch
Macaroni cheese p125
with halved cherry tomatoes
Mango lolly p132

Dinner
Salmon and dill risotto p186
with steamed sugar snaps
Apply plums p129

Saturday

Breakfast
Scrambled egg p99 with
buttered toast p69 and orange
segments

Lunch
Carrot and coriander soup p181
with savoury muffins p170
Rice pudding p135 with dried fruit

Dinner
Turkey and red pepper patties
p184 with peach chutney p182
and steamed green beans
Creamy apricot dessert p129

Sunday

Breakfast
Puffed rice cereal with milk
and banana slices

Lunch
Mini lamb and mint balls p109
with avocado dip p105 and
peppers
Mandarin jelly p192

Dinner
Garden vegetable risotto p127
Stewed plums p129

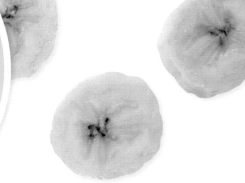

Other ideas this week Toast and peanut butter p101 and mango smoothie p171 • Broccoli cheese p125 with bread and butter • Ricotta, tomato, and basil sandwich p174 with carrot sticks • Chicken mini-burgers with fruity sauce p183 with green beans and bread • Yogurt and fruit

day-by-day meal planner
Week 9

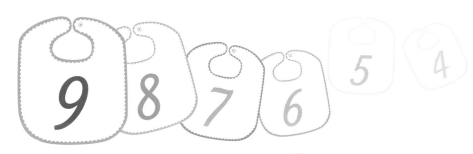

Monday

Breakfast
Fruits of the forest smoothie p168
with baby blueberry pancakes p169

Lunch
Cheesy tomato risotto p124
with steamed carrots
Stewed summer berries p191 and yogurt

Dinner
Chicken mini-burgers with fruity sauce
p183 with sweet potato and broccoli
Baked stuffed apple p190
and custard

Tuesday

Breakfast
Spicy banana toast p100 with sliced
strawberries or whole raspberries

Lunch
Mini lamb and mint balls p109 with
couscous p102, tzatziki, and cucumber
Segments of clementine or peach slices

Dinner
Vegetarian shepherd's pie p189 with
peas and steamed carrots
Exotic fruit salad p191

Wednesday

Breakfast
Puffed rice cereal with raisins
and milk and pear slices p130

Lunch
Baked beans on toast p173
Yogurt with berries

Dinner
Simple fish pie p187 with
sweetcorn and steamed
sugar snaps
Baked egg custard p195

Thursday

Breakfast
Simple muesli p169 with milk
and dried apple slices

Lunch
Creamy avocado pasta p188
with steamed broccoli fingers
Mango lolly p132

Dinner
Creamy vegetarian mince p126
with potato and parsnip or swede
Bread and butter pudding p194
with banana slices

Friday

Breakfast
Scrambled egg p99 with buttered
toast p69 and ready-to-eat apricots

Lunch
Pineapple and cheese on toast p173
with cucumber fingers
Semolina pudding p134 with
mashed berries

Dinner
Beef ragu p115 with pasta shapes
and steamed broccoli
Pear and raisin oat crumble p193

Saturday

Breakfast
Banana bread p168 with
cream cheese and halved grapes

Lunch
Sardines on toast p173
with red pepper and carrot sticks
Ground rice pudding p134
with mandarins

Dinner
Cauliflower or broccoli cheese p125
with bread and butter
Clementine or peach slices

Sunday

Breakfast
Raspberry porridge p99
with strawberry or mango slices

Lunch
Butternut or pumpkin and tomato soup
p180 with bread and butter fingers and
cubes of cheese
Mango smoothie p171

Dinner
Fruity chicken p112 with couscous p102
and steamed green beans
Pear and raisin oat crumble p193
with ice cream

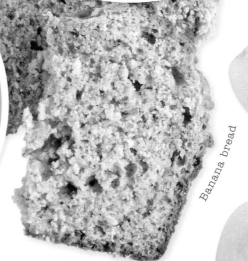

Banana bread

Other ideas this week Wheat biscuit with milk p70 and fruit • Pea and mint soup p181 with toast fingers • Mushroom and onion pizza p178 • Normandy pork p113 with potatoes and green beans • Crispy salmon fingers p186 with broccoli and potatoes • Chocolate rice pudding p135

day-by-day meal planner
Week 10

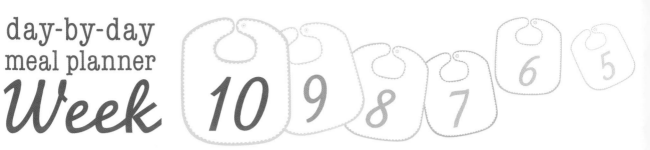

Monday

Breakfast
Scrambled egg p99 with buttered toast and orange segments

Lunch
Butternut or pumpkin and tomato soup p180 with tuna and avocado sandwich p175
Fromage frais with kiwi slices

Dinner
Vegetarian shepherd's pie p189 with steamed green beans
Baked spiced peach p190 with ice cream

Tuesday

Breakfast
Vanilla and banana smoothie p171 with sweetcorn and tomato fritter p172

Lunch
Baby falafel p110 with mashed potato, cooked spinach, and home-made tomato salsa p182
Yogurt or fromage frais

Dinner
Greek baked fish p120 with potato pieces and green beans
Chocolate rice pudding p135

Wednesday

Breakfast
Spicy plum and banana breakfast p96 with pear slices p130

Lunch
Tortilla with Mexican beans p177 with cucumber fingers
Fruits of the forest iced yogurt p133

Dinner
Bulghur wheat with lamb and aubergine p184 with steamed broccoli or courgette
Stewed apple and cranberries p129

Thursday

Breakfast
Bircher muesli p98 with strawberry or mango slices p131

Lunch
Ham and pineapple pizza p179 with pepper and carrot fingers
Pear or apple slices p130

Dinner
Beef meatballs in tomato sauce p185 with rice and steamed sugar snaps
Pancakes p192 with any fruit

Friday

Breakfast
Carrot muffin p171
with blueberries

Lunch
Salmon and dill risotto p186
with petit pois mixed in
Mango lolly p132

Dinner
Pork with pineapple p114 with rice,
peas, and steamed carrots
Canned pineapple chunks

Saturday

Breakfast
Puffed rice cereal with raisins, milk,
and banana slices

Lunch
Scrambled egg p99 with buttered toast
p69 and halved cherry tomatoes
Fromage frais with stewed apricots p129

Dinner
Shepherd's pie (with beef or lamb) p185
with steamed parsnip and courgette
Fruit fool p133

Sunday

Breakfast
Baked egg with cheese and tomato
p172 with bread and butter fingers

Lunch
Pea and mint soup p181
with savoury muffins p170
Fruit fool p133

Dinner
Chicken Provençale p112
with steamed potato and
broccoli pieces
Banana custard p133

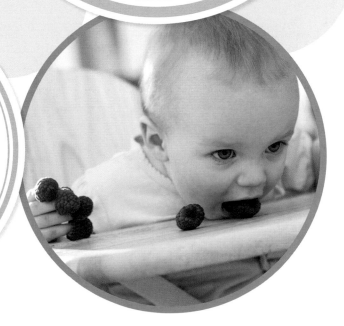

Other ideas this week Fromage frais with banana slices • Hard-boiled egg with buttered toast p69 • Pancake with cheese and tomato p177 • Simple fish pie p187 with green beans • Normandy pork p113 with potatoes and broccoli • Passion fruit and mango dessert p191

day-by-day meal planner Week

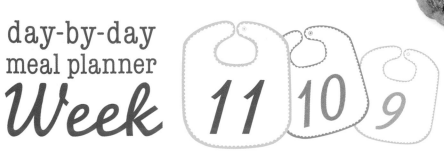

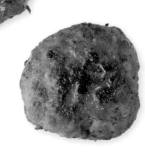

Monday

Breakfast
Bircher muesli p98
with blueberries or mango cubes

Lunch
Mini lamb and mint balls p109 with
couscous p102 and avocado dip p105
Banana custard p133

Dinner
Fruity chicken p112 with potato,
steamed cauliflower, and broccoli
Chocolate rice pudding p135

Tuesday

Breakfast
French toast p98 with currant bun
and ready-to-eat apricots, halved

Lunch
Beef with prunes p116 with sweet potato mash
and steamed broccoli
Stewed summer berries p191 and yogurt

Dinner
Bulghur wheat with currants
and chickpeas p187 with soft cooked
carrot and swede
Bread and butter
pudding p194

Wednesday

Breakfast
Puffed rice cereal with raisins, milk, and
clementine segments

Lunch
Pancakes p192 with salmon, yogurt, and
cucumber p176 with cucumber and
pepper fingers
Yogurt with berries

Dinner
Chicken and mushroom
casserole p113 with rice,
steamed broccoli, and carrots
Baked egg custard p195

Thursday

Breakfast
Buttered brioche slices, yogurt,
and raspberries or strawberries

Lunch
Creamy vegetarian mince p126
with pasta and steamed broccoli
Lemony ricotta pudding p134

Dinner
Turkey and red pepper patties
p184 with couscous p102, peach
chutney p182, and tomatoes
Exotic fruit salad p191

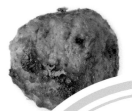

Friday

Breakfast
Date porridge p98
with kiwi slices

Lunch
Leek and potato soup p180
with egg and cress sandwich p175
Melon or mango cubes

Dinner
Shepherd's pie with beef p185 and peas
Baked spiced peach p190
with ice cream

Saturday

Breakfast
Apple yogurt breakfast with
ready-to-eat prunes, halved

Lunch
Pancake slices p192 with spicy
chicken and vegetables p176
Stewed plums p129 and custard

Dinner
Salmon and dill risotto p186 with
steamed green beans and broccoli
Pear and raisin oat crumble p193
with ice cream

Sunday

Breakfast
Scrambled egg p99 with buttered toast p69
and mango smoothie p171

Lunch
Pesto, tomato, and mozzarella pizza p178
with cucumber wedges
Pear or plum slices pp130–1

Dinner
Coconut lentil dhal p128 with naan bread
and steamed green beans
Exotic fruit salad p191

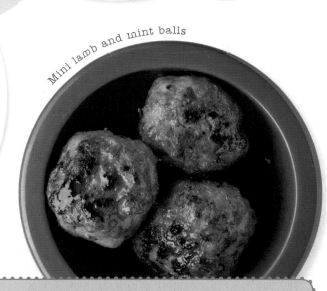

Mini lamb and mint balls

Other ideas this week Oat porridge p98 with fruit • Ricotta, tomato, and basil sandwich p174 with carrot and pepper sticks • Baked beans on toast p173 • Greek baked fish p120 with potatoes and cooked spinach • Creamy avocado pasta p188 with broccoli • Fruit fool p133

day-by-day meal planner

Week

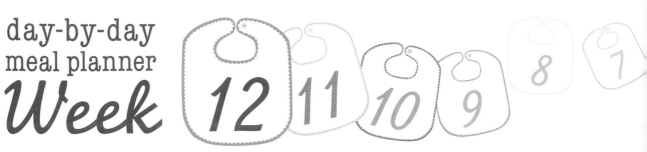

12 11 10 9 8 7

Monday

Breakfast
Simple muesli p169
with ready-to-eat apricots

Lunch
Crispy salmon fingers p186
with bread and butter, home-made
tomato salsa p182, and
cucumber fingers
Fromage frais with stewed fruit p129

Dinner
Shepherd's pie (lamb or beef) p185
with steamed sugar snaps and carrots
Lemony ricotta
pudding p134

Tuesday

Breakfast
Puffed rice cereal with raisins, milk,
and berries

Lunch
Pineapple and cheese on toast p173 with
halved cherry tomatoes and cucumber
Banana custard p133

Dinner
Creamy vegetable korma p126 with rice
and steamed broccoli
Mandarin jelly p192

Wednesday

Breakfast
French toast p98 with currant bun
and orange segments

Lunch
Scrambled egg p99 with halved cherry
tomatoes and bread and butter
Yogurt with berries

Dinner
Normandy pork p113 with potato mashed
with sweetcorn and steamed swede/parsnip
Rice pudding p135

Thursday

Breakfast
Vanilla and banana smoothie p171
with carrot muffin p171

Lunch
Sardines on toast p173
with cucumber fingers
Banana with chocolate dipping sauce p135

Dinner
Fruity chicken p112 with mashed
carrot and swede and pasta shapes
Yogurt

Friday

Breakfast
Cornflakes with milk
and banana slices

Lunch
Baby falafel p110 with tzatziki, pitta bread
strips, and tomato slices
Fruits of the forest iced yogurt p133

Dinner
Butternut squash risotto p122
with steamed green beans
Pancakes p192 with
stewed fruit p129

Saturday

Breakfast
Bircher muesli p98
with chopped prunes or figs

Lunch
Beef ragu p115 with cooked spinach and
pasta shapes
Exotic fruit salad p191

Dinner
Simple fish pie p187 with steamed sugar snaps
Stewed summer berries p191
and yogurt

Sunday

Breakfast
French toast p98 with currant bun
and clementine segments

Lunch
Cowboy beans with cornmeal topping p188
with steamed broccoli
Chocolate rice pudding p135

Dinner
Herby lamb with vegetables p114
with added peas and potato wedges
Baked stuffed apple p190 and custard

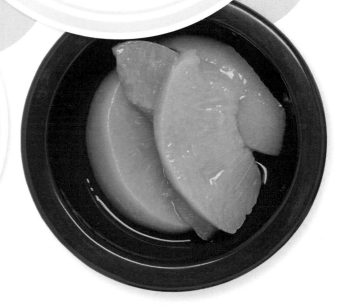

Other ideas this week Wheat biscuit with milk p70 and apricot purée p60 • Tuna and avocado sandwich p175 with red peppers • Carrot and coriander soup p181 with bread and butter • Beef ragu p115 with pasta and broccoli • Salmon and dill risotto p186 with green beans • Baked egg custard p195

day-by-day meal planner
Week 13

Monday

Breakfast
Spicy banana toast p100 with pear or apple slices p130

Lunch
Mackerel and tomato pizza p179 with carrot/pepper sticks
Mandarin jelly p192

Dinner
Shepherd's pie p185 with steamed carrots and sugar snaps
Blackberry apple cobbler p195

Tuesday

Breakfast
Baby blueberry pancakes p169 with butter and clementine segments

Lunch
White flaked fish p106, avocado dip p105, pitta strips, and cherry tomato pieces
Yogurt with berries

Dinner
Pork with pineapple p114 with rice, carrots, and peas
Bread and butter pudding p194

Wednesday

Breakfast
Banana bread p168 with cream cheese and berries

Lunch
Egg and cress sandwich p175 with halved grapes and clementine segments
Fruits of the forest smoothie p168

Dinner
Fruity chicken p112 with mashed sweet potato, steamed broccoli, and sugar snaps
Rice pudding p135 with kiwi slices

Thursday

Breakfast
Bircher muesli p98 with orange segments

Lunch
Cheesy tomato risotto p124 with steamed broccoli and carrots
Ready-to-eat apricots

Dinner
Beef ragu p115 with pasta shapes, spinach, and steamed carrots
Stewed summer berries p191 and yogurt

Friday

Breakfast
Scrambled egg p99 with buttered
toast p69 and berries

Lunch
Tortilla with Mexican beans p177
with cucumber pieces
Apple sponge pudding p193

Dinner
Turkey and red pepper patties p184
with roasted Mediterranean
vegetable dip p107 and bread
and butter
Exotic fruit salad p191

Saturday

Breakfast
Fruits of the forest smoothie p168
with savoury muffin p170

Lunch
Tuna and avocado sandwich p175
with cherry tomato pieces
Fromage frais with stewed fruit p129

Dinner
Vegetarian shepherd's pie p189
with steamed green vegetables
Pear and raisin oat
crumble p193 with ice cream

Sunday

Breakfast
Simple muesli p169
with strawberry or mango slices

Lunch
Carrot and coriander soup p181
with cheese scone p104
Banana slices with ice cream

Dinner
Beef meatballs in tomato sauce
p185 with mashed peas and potato
Apricot and almond pudding p194

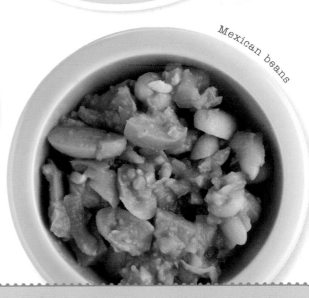

Mexican beans

Other ideas this week French toast with fruit p98 • Baked potato with cheese and tomato p177 • Ham and pineapple pizza p179 • Crispy salmon fingers p186 with mashed peas • Creamy avocado pasta p188 with broccoli • Baked stuffed apple p190

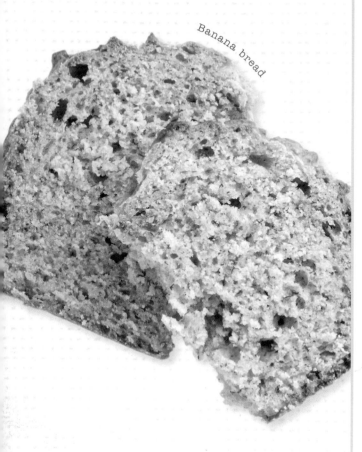

Banana bread

Banana bread

Many banana bread recipes are really cakes, but this one doesn't use sugar, relying instead on the sweetness of the ripe banana.

 5 mins   30–35 mins   8 baby portions

ingredients

50ml (1¾fl oz) **vegetable oil**, plus extra for greasing
2 large ripe **bananas** or 200g (7oz) after peeling

2 large **eggs**
1 tsp **vanilla extract**
125g (4½oz) **plain flour**
125g (4½oz) **wholemeal flour**
2 tsp **baking powder**

method

1 Preheat the oven to 190°C (375°F/Gas 5). Lightly oil a 900g (2lb) loaf tin.

2 Mash the bananas until smooth and place in a mixing bowl. Stir in the oil, eggs, and vanilla extract.

3 Sieve the flours and baking powder, adding back any that stays in the sieve.

4 Stir the dry ingredients into the wet mixture and beat together until smooth. Pour or spoon into the prepared tin and bake for 30–35 minutes, or until risen and lightly browned.

5 Cool on a wire rack, then slice, and store.

✳ **Serve** *with cream cheese, butter or spread.*
✳ **Refrigerate** *or freeze on the day of making when cooled.*

Fruits of the forest smoothie

Berries, currants, and cherries all fall under this lovely name, so choose whichever fruits you and your baby particularly enjoy and are in season. In winter, you can use frozen berries, either individually, or look out for packets that have a fruits of the forest mix.

 5 mins   1–2 baby portions

ingredients

100g (3½oz) **berries** and/or **currants**, such as **blueberries, strawberries, cherries, black currants** or **red currants**
75g (2½oz) **plain yogurt**

method

1 If using fresh fruits, remove the stalks and wipe with damp kitchen paper.

2 Process the ingredients until smooth.

3 Serve half of it straight away in a beaker and chill the remainder.

✳ **Serve** *for breakfast.*
✳ **Refrigerate** *in an airtight container for 24 hours.*

Baby blueberry pancakes

Blueberry pancakes are a breakfast staple in the US, providing a little fruit inside a delicious pancake that your baby can eat with his fingers. The fruit usually softens easily during the cooking process, but if you are concerned about it being a choking hazard, you can process it a little to make a purple pancake batter.

 5 mins 10–15 mins 4 baby and 4 adult portions ❄

ingredients

1 **egg**
175ml (6fl oz) **buttermilk**,
  or 100g (3½oz) **plain
  yogurt** and 80ml (2¾fl oz)
  whole milk
100g (3½oz) **self-raising flour**
1 tsp **baking powder**
1 tbsp **maple syrup**
  or 2 tsp **sugar**
1 tsp **vanilla extract**
150g (5½oz) **blueberries**
1 tbsp **vegetable oil**,
  for greasing

method

1 Preheat a griddle or non-stick frying pan over a medium–high heat.

2 Blend all the ingredients, except the blueberries, until smooth. Then stir in the blueberries.

3 Brush the pan or griddle lightly with oil and spoon a few dessertspoonfuls of batter into the pan. For adult pancakes, use 2–3 dessertspoonfuls and 1 for baby pancakes. Cook the pancakes on one side, then carefully turn over to cook on the other side.

4 When cooked on both sides, remove from the pan. Repeat the process with the remaining batter. Allow to cool a little before serving or storing.

✳ **Serve** *with cream cheese or a fruit purée (see pp59–62).*
✳ **Refrigerate** *in an airtight container for 24 hours or freeze.*
✳ **Variations:** *When apricots are in season, replace the blueberries with chopped fresh apricots.*

Simple muesli

Rather than sugar-coated breakfast cereals, why not make this easy muesli for your baby? It provides essential iron and fibre and stores for a few days.

 5 mins   4 baby portions

ingredients

50g (1¾oz) **rolled oats**
10g (¼oz) **ground
  almonds**
10g (¼oz) **dessicated
  coconut**

50g (1¾oz) ready-to-eat
  apricots, chopped
  very finely.

method

1 Mix all the ingredients together and store in an airtight container.

2 Serve with whole milk or plain yogurt.

✳ **Serve** *with a few slices of banana.*
✳ **Store** *in an airtight container for up to 3–4 days.*
✳ **Variations:** *Apricots can be replaced with any dried fruit of your choice, including dried prunes, raisins or dates. Chop them well as raisins can cause choking, especially if not softened.*

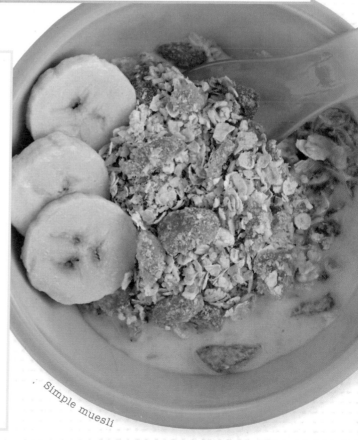

Simple muesli

Savoury muffins

Breakfast muffins don't need to be full of sugar, and this version sneaks in courgettes and cheese for a delicious starchy start to the day. They can also be served with soup or make a tasty snack. Conveniently, they freeze well.

 10 mins 12–20 mins 6 baby and 6 adult portions

ingredients

75g (2½oz) **plain flour**
75g (2½oz) **wholemeal flour**
3 tsp **baking powder**
100g (3½oz) **courgette**, finely grated
60g (2oz) **hard cheese**, grated
1 tbsp finely chopped herbs such as **parsley, oregano** or **marjoram** (optional)
1 **egg**
100ml (3½fl oz) **whole milk**
2 tbsp **vegetable oil**

method

1 Preheat the oven to 200°C (400°F/Gas 6). Grease a mini muffin and standard muffin tray, or line with muffin cases.

2 Sieve the flours together with the baking powder into a mixing bowl, adding back any bran that remains in the sieve afterwards.

3 Add the courgette, cheese, and herbs, if using.

4 Beat the egg in a bowl and stir in the milk and oil. Pour these over the dry ingredients to make a thick mixture.

5 Spoon the mixture into the muffin cases or tray. Bake for 12–15 minutes for the smaller muffins and 18–20 minutes for the larger ones.

✳ **Serve** *at breakfast with diluted fruit juice, eggs or fresh fruit pieces.*
✳ **Refrigerate** *for up to 48 hours or freeze when cool.*

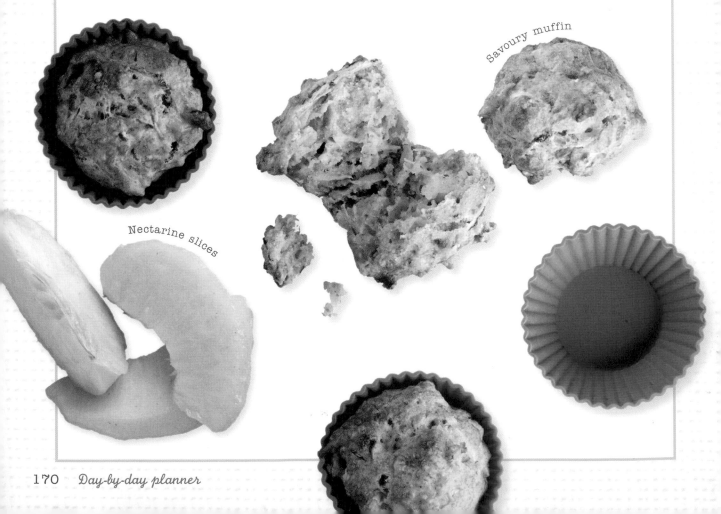

Nectarine slices

Savoury muffin

Carrot muffins

These light muffins provide essential calcium for a great start to the day. As with the savoury muffins, these can be enjoyed at any time of the day and make a good transportable meal for days out.

 10 mins   12–15 mins   12 baby muffins

ingredients

2 tbsp **vegetable oil**, plus extra for greasing
125g (4½oz) **self-raising flour**
1 **egg**
100ml (3½fl oz) **whole milk**
60g (2oz) **carrots**, grated
50g (1¾oz) **hard cheese**, grated

method

1 Preheat the oven to 200°C (400°F/Gas 6). Grease a mini muffin tray or line with mini muffin cases.

2 Sieve the flour into a bowl and add the egg, milk, and oil. Beat together with a blender or whisk to make a thick batter. Stir in the carrots and cheese.

3 Spoon the mixture into the muffin cases or tray and bake for 12–15 minutes, or until golden brown.

✳ **Serve** *at breakfast with diluted fruit juice, eggs or fresh fruit pieces.*
✳ **Refrigerate** *for up to 48 hours or freeze when cool.*

Mango smoothie

Mangoes make a delicious smoothie that provides essential vitamin C. Serve to your baby in a lidded beaker for him to sip.

 5 mins   4 baby portions

ingredients

½ ripe **mango**, cut into cubes, or 150g (5½oz) mango cubes

100ml (3½fl oz) unsweetened **pineapple** or **apple juice**

method

1 Blend the mango cubes and juice until smooth.

2 Chill until required.

✳ **Serve** *in a beaker as part of a main meal.*
✳ **Refrigerate** *in an airtight container for up to 24 hours.*
✳ **Variations:** *Add a ripe peach or nectarine, skinned and chopped, in step 1.*

Vanilla and banana smoothie

Breakfast in a beaker for your baby, this easy-to-make, calcium-rich smoothie is bound to be popular.

 5 mins   1 baby portion

ingredients

½ ripe **banana**, cut into chunks
75g (2½oz) **plain yogurt**

1–2 drops **vanilla extract**

method

1 Blend the banana, yogurt, and vanilla extract until smooth.

2 Serve in a beaker straight away.

✳ **Serve** *as an accompaniment to a main meal.*
✳ *Not suitable for storage.*
✳ **Variations:** *Add 1–2 ready-to-eat chopped apricots.*

Baked egg with cheese and tomato

Oven-baked eggs make a nice change to hard-boiled ones, and your baby will enjoy the variety of flavours here.

 5 mins   10 mins 1 baby portion

ingredients

vegetable oil, for greasing
½ **tomato**, halved, deseeded, and finely chopped
1 **egg**
10g (¼oz) **Cheddar cheese**, grated

method

1 Preheat the oven to 180°C (350°F/Gas 4). Lightly grease a small ovenproof dish, such as a ramekin.

2 Place the tomato at the base of the dish and crack the egg over it.

3 Sprinkle with the cheese, and bake uncovered for around 10 minutes, or until the yolk has set.

✳ **Serve** *with pieces of buttered toast or bread.*
✳ *Not suitable for storage.*
✳ **Variations:** *Add a few chopped chives or a small quantity of shredded ham.*

Sweetcorn and tomato fritters

These little fritters make a lovely weekend breakfast when you may have a bit more time to cook. It won't be just your baby enjoying them – you'll love them, too. By this stage, your baby will be able to cope with lumps so the sweetcorn shouldn't be a problem. If he is slow to chew, you can pulse the sweetcorn a little in a processor.

 5 mins   5–10 mins   20 fritters

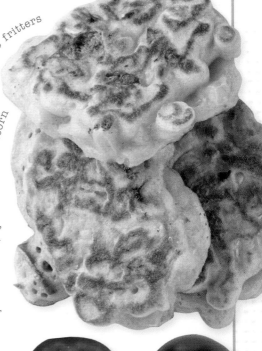

Sweetcorn and tomato fritters

ingredients

100g (3½oz) **self-raising flour**
1 **egg**
150ml (5fl oz) **whole milk**
1–2 tsp chopped **chives**
1 medium **tomato**, halved, deseeded and finely chopped
150g (5½oz) **sweetcorn kernels**, canned in water, or frozen and defrosted
1–2 tbsp **vegetable oil**

method

1 Make the batter by blending the flour, egg, and milk until smooth.

2 Pour into a bowl or jug, and add the chives, tomato, and sweetcorn. Stir well to combine.

3 Heat 1 tablespoon of the oil in a large non-stick frying pan. Spoon around 1 tablespoon of the batter into the hot oil, and repeat until you have several fritters cooking.

4 Fry for 2–4 minutes, or until golden brown at the base, then turn over and cook on the other side. Drain on kitchen paper and continue cooking until all the batter is used up.

✳ **Serve** *with a few halved cherry tomatoes.*
✳ **Wrap** *individually in cling film and refrigerate for 24 hours or freeze when cooled.*

Sardines on toast

Sardines are fantastically nutritious – high in zinc, iron, and B vitamins, and the soft bones provide calcium and vitamin D. Mash well to incorporate the bones.

 2 mins    3 mins   1 baby portion

ingredients

1 slice **bread**
  of your choice
1 canned **sardine** in oil
  or tomato sauce
1 tsp **lemon juice** (optional)
cucumber slices

method

1 Preheat the grill and toast the bread on both sides.

2 Mash the canned sardine well with the lemon juice, if using.

3 Spread over the toast and grill for 2–3 minutes, or until bubbling and hot.

4 Cool and cut into pieces. Serve with cucumber slices.

✷ Note: *Mackerel or pilchards can be used instead of sardines. These oily fish retain their omega 3 during the canning process, unlike tuna.*

Pineapple and cheese on toast

Pineapple and cheese is a delicious combination. Canned pineapple in juice is softer than the fresh fruit, so easier for babies to chew – and available whatever the season.

 2 mins   3 mins   1 baby portion

ingredients

1 slice **bread** of your choice
1 tsp **butter** or **olive spread**
1 canned **pineapple ring** in juice,
  plus more to serve
15g (½oz) **Cheddar cheese**, grated

method

1 Preheat the grill. Toast the bread, and spread with the butter or olive spread.

2 Cut the pineapple into small chunks and scatter over the toast. Then sprinkle over the cheese.

3 Grill for 2–3 minutes, or until the cheese is bubbling and brown.

4 Remove from the heat, cool slightly, and cut into pieces. Serve with more chunks of pineapple.

Baked beans on toast

Did you know that baked beans combined with wheat toast provides a great mix of proteins for vegetarian babies? Not only that, but the beans provide iron, too. Choose salt- and sugar-reduced varieties of baked beans.

 2 mins   3 mins   1 baby portion

ingredients

1 heaped tbsp **baked beans**
1 slice **bread** of your choice
1 tsp **butter** or **olive spread**

method

1 Heat the beans in a saucepan or microwave oven until they are piping hot. Pour into a little bowl, and allow to cool to body temperature.

2 Meanwhile, toast the bread, and spread with the butter or olive spread.

3 Cut the toast into pieces and serve with the beans.

Ways with *sandwiches*

Sandwiches make a simply prepared meal that's both portable and easy for your baby to pick up. Your baby may manage one slice of bread cut in half and sandwiched together, or want more or less than this, depending on her appetite. Choose nutritious fillings that provide protein as well as vegetables. It doesn't matter if your baby has white, wholemeal or half-and-half bread at this stage; in fact, it is a good idea to let her sample these different varieties now, then by one year she can branch out more and try breads with grains or seeds.

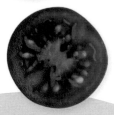

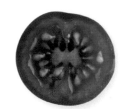

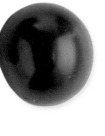

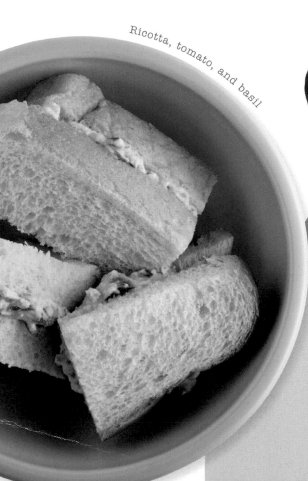

Ricotta, tomato, and basil

Ricotta, tomato, and basil

ingredients

1 heaped tbsp **ricotta cheese**

½ **tomato**, deseeded and finely chopped

2 small **basil leaves**, shredded

1 slice **bread** of your choice

carrot or cucumber, cut into batons, to serve

method

1 Mix the ricotta and tomato together, then add the basil.

2 Spread these over the bread, and cut in half.

3 Sandwich together, cut into small pieces or quarters, and serve the sandwiches with the carrot or cucumber batons.

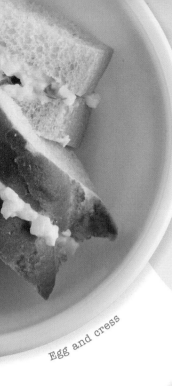

Egg and cress

Egg and cress

ingredients

1 **egg**
1 tbsp reduced-fat **mayonnaise**
1 slice **bread** of your choice
1 tbsp **cress**, finely chopped
cherry tomatoes, halved,
   to serve

* *Extra egg mixture can be refrigerated in an airtight container overnight.*

method

1 Hard boil the egg by cooking in a saucepan of simmering water for up to 10 minutes. Remove and cool by dipping into cold water. Shell the egg and chop into a bowl.

2 Stir in the mayonnaise and mix well to combine. Spread over the bread, then sprinkle over the cress, and cut in half.

3 Sandwich together, cut into small pieces or quarters, and serve with the cherry tomatoes.

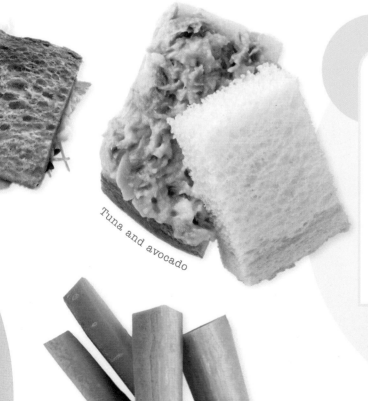

Tuna and avocado

Tuna and avocado

ingredients

½ small **avocado**
1 tsp **lemon** or **lime juice**
25g (scant 1oz) **canned
   tuna** in oil or water

1 slice **bread** of your
   choice
cherry tomatoes,
   halved, to serve

method

1 Scoop the avocado into a small bowl, sprinkle with the lemon juice, and mash until soft.

2 Stir in the tuna and mix well. Spread over the bread, and cut in half.

3 Sandwich together, cut into small pieces or quarters, and serve with the cherry tomatoes.

Ways with *fillers*

For babies approaching one year old, self-feeding becomes less tricky, even if the mess is the same. Filled pancakes, tortillas, and chapattis provide a new experience, and can be eaten as finger foods. These fillings can also be used in baked potatoes. Here is a variety of toppings; on page 192 there is a pancake recipe that can be batch-cooked and frozen.

Salmon, yogurt, and cucumber

A summery filling to use either cold or at room temperature, salmon provides essential omega 3 fatty acids.

5 mins   12–15 mins   6 baby portions

ingredients

60g (2oz) cooked **salmon** (see p186)
2 heaped tbsp **full-fat plain yogurt**
½ tsp finely grated **lemon zest**
3cm (1in) piece **cucumber**, finely chopped

method

1 Check the cooked salmon for bones and flake into a small bowl. Stir in the yogurt, lemon zest, and cucumber.

2 Chill until required or use straight away.

✳ *Not suitable for freezing. Must be eaten chilled within 24 hours.*

✳ **Variation:** *Replace the cucumber with ¹/₂ small avocado, cut into small cubes.*

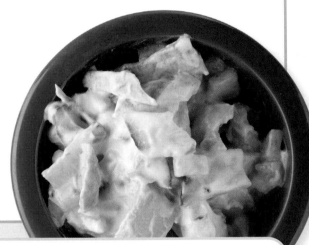

Spicy chicken and vegetables

Fill tortillas or pancakes and slice as finger food or serve the chicken in a bowl with pieces of pancake or tortilla on the side.

5 mins   20–25 mins   6 baby portions

ingredients

1 tbsp **olive** or **vegetable oil**
1 small **onion**, finely chopped
100g (3½oz) **chicken breast fillets**, roughly chopped
¼ **red pepper**, sliced
100g (3½oz) **mushrooms**, sliced
200g (7oz) canned chopped **tomatoes** in juice
pinch of **Cajun spices** (optional)

method

1 Heat the oil in a non-stick saucepan and fry the onion and chicken, stirring frequently, until the chicken is lightly coloured on all sides.

2 Add all the remaining ingredients and gently bring to a simmering point. Stir, cover, and continue cooking for 15–20 minutes until the vegetables are tender. Cool a little before using.

✳ **Refrigerate** *for 24 hours or freeze when cooled.*

✳ **Variations:** *Use 100g (3¹/₂oz) courgette instead of the mushrooms. For the adult portion, add more Cajun spices.*

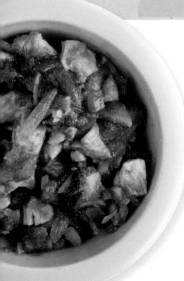

Cheese and tomato

Simply cooked onion and tomato with a little cheese provides protein and vitamin C and makes a popular filling for tortillas. It can be varied in many ways.

 5 mins 15 mins 2–3 baby portions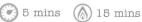

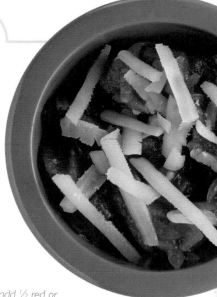

ingredients

1 tbsp **olive** or **vegetable oil**
1 small **onion**, finely chopped
200g (7oz) fresh **tomatoes**, roughly chopped
pinch of **thyme**
15g (½oz) **Cheddar cheese**, grated (for each pancake, baked potato, or tortilla)

method

1 Heat the oil in a small saucepan and gently fry the onion for about 5 minutes, or until lightly browned and slightly softened, stirring frequently.

2 Add the chopped tomatoes and thyme and cook over a medium heat for 10 minutes, stirring frequently, until the mixture is thickened and the tomatoes soft. Cool slightly.

3 Serve, sprinkled with the grated cheese.

✳ Refrigerate *for 24 hours or freeze when cooled.*

✳ Variations: *Use 200g (7oz) chopped canned tomatoes instead of the fresh tomatoes. You can also add ½ red or green pepper, finely chopped, or 50g (1¾oz) mushrooms, finely sliced.*

Mexican beans

Beans are a good source of B vitamins and iron. Pinto beans are usually used in this dish, but other beans such as cannellini or black-eyed beans are good, too. Canned beans save time. Buy ones canned in water with no salt.

 5–10 mins 25–30 mins 2 adult and 2 baby portions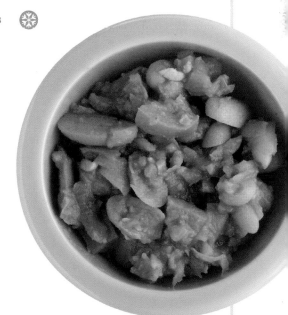

ingredients

2 tbsp **olive oil**
100g (3½oz) or 1 medium **onion**, finely sliced
2 **garlic cloves**, crushed
160g (5¾oz), or 1 **red** or **orange pepper**, diced
1 tsp **ground cumin**
400g (14oz) can **beans** in water, drained
60g (2oz) or 2 heaped tbsp **tomato purée**

For adult portions:
Tabasco sauce, to your taste
1–2 tbsp **jalapeno peppers**, chopped

method

1 Heat the oil in a non-stick saucepan and gently fry the onion and garlic for 5 minutes, or until softened.

2 Stir in the pepper and cumin and continue cooking for another few minutes, stirring continuously. Add the beans, tomato purée, and 300ml (10fl oz) water, and bring to the boil.

3 Stir, cover, and simmer for 15–20 minutes, or until the vegetables are tender. Take off the heat and cool a little.

4 Remove about 3 rounded tablespoons per portion for your baby and process roughly to achieve a suitable texture. Allow to cool more while you add the Tabasco and jalapenos to your portion.

✳ Refrigerate *in an airtight container for up to 24 hours or freeze when cooled.*

Ways with *pizzas*

Make your own pizza toppings for your baby's light meals using fresh ingredients. A halved English muffin makes a great base, but you could of course use a thick slice of bread or a halved bread roll.

⏱ 5 mins   🔥 6–8 mins   ◔ 1–2 baby portions

Pesto, tomato, and mozzarella

ingredients

½ **English muffin**
½ tsp **pesto**
3 **cherry tomatoes**, finely chopped
15g (½oz) **mozzarella cheese**, diced

✳ *Serve with carrot, pepper or cucumber batons.*

✳ *Not suitable for storing.*

✳ **Tip:** *Pesto is salty, so use just a little. You can also replace the pesto with 1 teaspoon of tomato purée.*

method

1 Preheat the oven to 220°C (425°F/Gas 7). Spread the muffin with the pesto. Cover with the tomatoes and mozzarella cheese.

2 Place on a baking sheet and bake for 5–7 minutes, or until the cheese is melted and just browning. Cool before cutting into pieces for your baby.

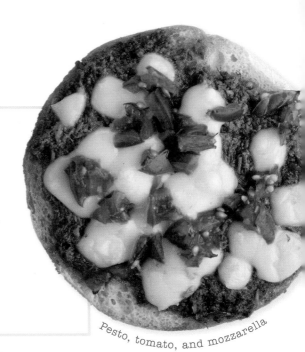

Pesto, tomato, and mozzarella

Mushroom and onion

ingredients

1 tsp **olive oil**
1 medium **mushroom**, finely chopped
2 **onion** slices, finely chopped

2 tsp **tomato purée**
pinch of dried **oregano**
½ **English muffin**
15g (½oz) **Cheddar cheese**, grated

method

1 Preheat the oven to 220°C (425°F/Gas 7).

2 Place the oil, mushroom, and onion in a small bowl and cover with cling film. Pierce with a knife before cooking on high for 40–50 seconds in a microwave oven to soften.

3 Cool a little, and stir in the tomato purée and oregano. Spread over the muffin and sprinkle over the cheese.

4 Place on a baking sheet and bake for 5–7 minutes, or until the cheese is melted and just browning. Cool before cutting into pieces for your baby.

✳ *Serve with carrot, pepper or cucumber batons.*

✳ *Not suitable for storing.*

✳ **Note:** *It is easier to cook the mushroom and onion mix in the microwave in a small bowl since the amount is little, but you can also soften on the hob in a small saucepan, if you prefer.*

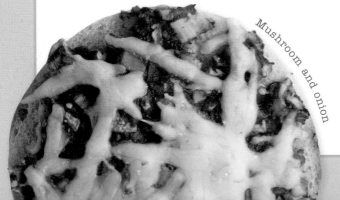

Mushroom and onion

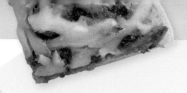

Mackerel and tomato

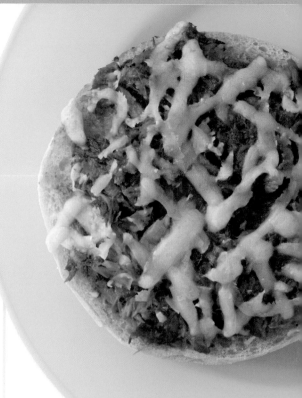

ingredients

- 2 tsp **tomato purée**
- 1 tsp **lemon juice**
- 20g (¾oz) canned **mackerel fillets**, steamed, or canned in oil
- ½ **English muffin**
- 15g (½oz) **Cheddar cheese**, grated

✱ *Serve with carrot, pepper or cucumber batons.*

✱ *Not suitable for storing.*

✱ *Note: Canned fish may be quite salty, so look out for mackerel fillets with the least salt. These may be steamed natural fillets or fillets canned in oil or tomato sauce, rather than brine. If using fillets in tomato sauce, there is no need to add the tomato purée.*

method

1 Preheat the oven to 220°C (425°F/Gas 7).

2 Mash together the tomato purée, lemon juice, and mackerel. Spread over the muffin and sprinkle with the cheese.

3 Place on a baking sheet and bake for 5–7 minutes, or until the cheese is bubbling and golden brown. Cool before cutting into small pieces for your baby.

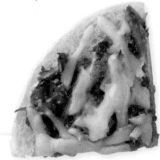

Mackerel and tomato

Ham and pineapple

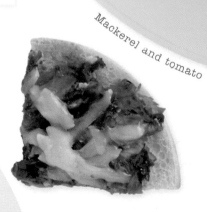

ingredients

- ½ **English muffin**
- 1 tsp **tomato purée**
- 10g (¼oz) unsmoked **ham** slice
- 1 slice **canned pineapple** in juice, finely chopped, or 1 tbsp drained crushed pineapple
- 15g (½oz) **Cheddar cheese**, grated

✱ *Serve with carrot, pepper or cucumber batons.*

✱ *Not suitable for storing.*

✱ *Tip: Ham can be very salty, so use only the quantity suggested, and choose unsmoked ham or reduced-salt ham, if available.*

method

1 Preheat the oven to 220°C (425°F/Gas 7).

2 Spread the muffin with the tomato purée and place the ham on top. Spread the pineapple over the top and sprinkle with the cheese.

3 Place on a baking sheet and bake for 5–7 minutes, or until the cheese is bubbling and golden brown. Cool before cutting into small pieces for your baby.

Leek and potato soup

Homely and filling, leek and potato soup always hits the spot on a cold day, so get your baby used to eating this mildly flavoured soup. Use reduced-salt stock, or water, and then season your own portion at the table. Leeks supply the B vitamin folate as well as plant substances called polyphenols that protect the body from disease.

 10 mins   15–20 mins 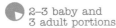 2–3 baby and 3 adult portions

ingredients

2 tbsp **vegetable oil**

3 or 500g (1lb 2oz) **leeks**, trimmed, washed, and sliced

500g (1lb 2oz) **floury potatoes**, peeled and diced

1 litre (1¾ pints) well-diluted low-salt **vegetable** or **chicken stock**

1 tbsp **chives**, chopped

For each adult serving, add 1 heaped tsp **crème fraîche** or reduced-fat **soured cream**

method

1 Heat the oil in a large non-stick saucepan and fry the leeks and potatoes for 5 minutes, stirring continuously.

2 Add the stock and bring to the boil. Cover and simmer for 10–15 minutes, or until the potatoes are tender. Add half the chives and purée until smooth.

3 Remove your baby's portion and allow to cool to lukewarm.

4 Season the adult portions and serve with the crème fraîche or soured cream, and the remaining chives.

✱ **Serve** with Cheesy polenta twigs (see p108) or Cheese scones (see p104).

✱ **Refrigerate** in an airtight container for up to 48 hours, or freeze on day of cooking when cooled.

Butternut or pumpkin and tomato soup

Pumpkin or other squashes can be roasted easily, which brings out their natural sweetness. Butternut squash is a significantly better source of vitamin A than pumpkin.

 10 mins   45–50 mins 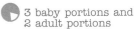 3 baby portions and 2 adult portions

ingredients

300g (10½oz) prepared **butternut squash** or **pumpkin**, cut into large chunks

1 large **red onion**, peeled and quartered

250g (9oz) ripe **tomatoes**, halved

1 sprig of **rosemary**

2 tbsp **olive oil**

400ml (14fl oz) low-salt **vegetable stock**

pinch of **nutmeg**, to serve (optional)

2 tbsp **crème fraîche** to serve

method

1 Preheat the oven to 200°C (400°F/Gas 6).

2 Place the squash or pumpkin, onion, tomatoes, and rosemary in a roasting tin and drizzle over the oil. Give the pan a good shake to mix the vegetables with the oil.

3 Roast for 40–45 minutes, or until the vegetables are softened. Remove from the oven and cool a little.

4 Purée half the vegetables with half the stock until smooth. Pour through a sieve over a clean saucepan, then repeat the process with the remaining vegetables and stock.

5 Check the seasoning, adding a little nutmeg, if desired. Serve warm with a swirl of crème fraîche on top.

✱ **Serve** with bread and butter pieces or home-made croutons (see below).

✱ **Refrigerate** for up to 48 hours or freeze on the day of cooking when cooled.

✱ **Make simple healthier croutons:** While the vegetables are roasting, cut 2 slices of any bread into 1cm (½in) cubes. Place on a baking sheet, spray with an oil mister, and bake for 10 minutes, turning once.

Carrot and coriander soup

This classic soup is full of vitamin A, and your baby will enjoy dipping in bread crusts, pitta bread or the Cheesy polenta twigs (see p108).

 10 mins   25–30 mins 6–8 baby and 2–3 adult portions

ingredients

2 tbsp **olive oil**
1 medium **onion**, roughly chopped
1 **garlic clove**, crushed
750g (1lb 10oz) **carrots**, scrubbed and roughly grated
1.5 litres (2½ pints) **water** or diluted low-salt **vegetable stock**
1 tsp **ground coriander**
2 tbsp **chopped coriander**
1 tsp **single cream**, to serve (optional)

method

1 Heat the oil in a large saucepan and gently fry the onion and garlic for about 5 minutes.

2 Add the carrots, stir, cover, and sweat for 5 more minutes, or until softened but not browned.

3 Add the stock and ground coriander, and bring to the boil. Stir, cover, and simmer for 15–20 minutes, or until the vegetables are soft.

4 Remove from the heat and stir in the fresh coriander. Blend the soup in batches until you have a smooth soup, being careful as the hot soup can scald.

5 Cool until just warm, and serve a ladleful to your baby in a beaker with a handle to drink, or in a shallow bowl. Stir in the cream to serve, if desired.

✱ Serve *with Cheesy polenta twigs (see p108), Cheese scones (see p104) or bread/toast pieces.*
✱ Refrigerate *for 48 hours or freeze on the day of cooking when cooled.*
✱ Note: *For adults, season with a little salt and black pepper.*

Pea and mint soup

This nutritious pea soup has to be one of the easiest to make, and knocks spots off any bought soup! Rich in vitamin C and fibre, it is on the table in less than 20 minutes. An older baby can drink it from a cup; younger ones may enjoy dipping in bread fingers or cheese scones.

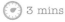 3 mins   10–12 mins   2 baby and 3 adult portions

ingredients

1 tbsp **vegetable oil**
1 medium **onion**, chopped
500g (1lb 2oz) **frozen peas**
600ml (1 pint) low-salt

vegetable stock
3–4 **mint leaves**
black pepper and **freshly grated nutmeg**, to serve

method

1 Heat the oil in a non-stick saucepan, and fry the onion gently until softened.

2 Add the peas and stock, and bring to the boil. Simmer for 5 minutes, or until the peas are just tender.

3 Add the mint leaves and then remove the soup from the heat.

5 Cool slightly before blending until smooth. Season with the black pepper and nutmeg, and serve.

✱ Serve *with a swirl of cream, if desired, Cheese scones (see p104) or bread and butter pieces.*

✱ Refrigerate *in an airtight container for up to 24 hours or freeze on the day of cooking when cooled.*

✱ Variations: *Add 2 handfuls of washed spinach in step 2 to provide additional iron and folate. For a creamier soup, replace half the stock with whole milk.*

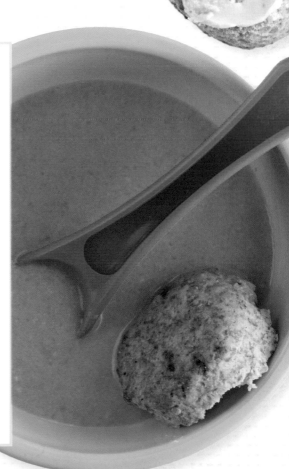

Home-made tomato salsa

Shop-bought salsa usually has salt and chilli, which aren't suitable for babies, so making your own with fresh ingredients gives you control over what to add, and home-made usually provides more vitamin C than shop-bought. It will still taste quite strong because of the raw onion, which some babies don't enjoy, so you may want to try with a little less onion at first.

 10 mins   2 baby and 2 adult portions

ingredients

1 tbsp or 250g (9oz) ripe **tomatoes**, washed and halved

½ small **onion**, peeled and quartered, or 3 **spring onions**, trimmed and quartered

½ small **red pepper**, roughly chopped (optional)

1 **garlic clove**, crushed

5g (⅛oz) fresh **coriander**

1 tbsp **lemon juice**

black pepper

method

1 Blend all the ingredients and pulse until they are roughly chopped. Be careful not to over-process them.

✱ **Serve** *with Turkey and red pepper patties (see p184), breadsticks, batons of carrots or other vegetables.*

✱ **Refrigerate** *in an airtight container for up to 24 hours.*

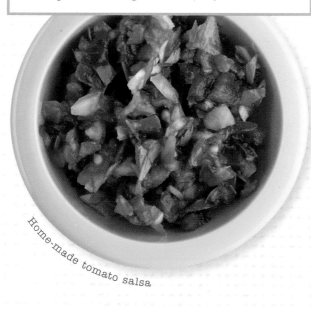

Home-made tomato salsa

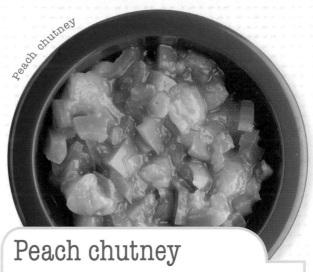

Peach chutney

Peach chutney

This is an easy fresh chutney that makes a great accompaniment to simply cooked foods, especially chicken or turkey burgers or fillets. When fresh peaches are in season use these, but otherwise you can use peaches canned in juice.

 5 mins 6 baby or 1 baby and 2 adult portions

 15–20 mins ❄

ingredients

2 tsp **vegetable oil**

½ small **onion**, finely chopped

45g (1½oz) **yellow** or **orange pepper**, deseeded and diced

1 ripe **peach**, skinned, stoned, and finely chopped, or 100g (3½oz) **canned peach** in juice

2 tbsp **water** or **juice**, if using canned peaches

1 tsp **wine vinegar**

1 tsp **demerara sugar**

method

1 Heat the oil in a small non-stick saucepan and gently fry the onion and peppers for 5 minutes, or until softened but not browned.

2 Add the peach, water or juice, vinegar, and sugar, and bring to the boil. Stir, reduce the heat, cover, and simmer for 10 minutes, or until the mixture has thickened.

3 Cool to room temperature and serve.

✱ **Serve** *with Turkey and red pepper patties (see p184), Chicken burgers (see opposite) or Crispy salmon fingers (see p186).*

✱ **Refrigerate** *up to 24 hours or freeze on cooking day when cool.*

✱ **Tip:** *To skin a peach, score a cross at the base and place in a heat-proof bowl. Cover with boiling water and leave for 20 seconds. Remove with a perforated spoon or tongs, and peel.*

Chicken mini-burgers with fruity sauce

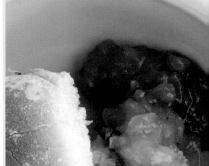

Chicken mini-burgers

A can of apricots in juice makes a sweet sauce to accompany these Thai-style mini-burgers. You can add chopped red chilli or Tabasco to your portion.

 10–15 mins 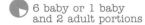 15 mins   6 baby or 1 baby and 2 adult portions

ingredients

250g (9oz) **chicken mince** (or process skinless **chicken breast** in a blender)
1 small **garlic clove**, crushed
1 tsp **lemongrass paste**
½ small **onion**, finely chopped
1 tbsp chopped **coriander**

For the sauce:
200g (7oz) can **apricot halves** in juice
½ small **onion**, finely chopped
30g (1oz) **golden raisins** or **sultanas**
1 tsp **lime juice**
finely grated zest of ½ **lime**

method

1 For the sauce, drain the apricot juice and reserve it. Place 120g (4¼oz) of the apricots in a small sacepan with the onion, raisins, and 60ml (2fl oz) of the reserved juice.

2 Bring the sauce to the boil, stir, cover, and simmer for 10–15 minutes, stirring occasionally to break up the apricots. Preheat a grill or griddle pan.

3 Meanwhile, place all the burger ingredients in a bowl and mix to combine well. Divide into about 6 little patties, and flatten to 1–2cm (½–¾in) thickness.

4 Grill or griddle for 3–4 minutes on each side, or until the meat is cooked through and the juices run clear, not pink, when pierced with a knife.

5 When the sauce is thickened, add the lime juice and zest; remove from the heat. For a lumpier sauce, mash; for a smoother sauce, blend briefly. Cool before serving.

✳ **Serve** *with mini-bread rolls and green or salad vegetables, either raw or steamed as appropriate.*

✳ *The sauce and burgers can be refrigerated for 24 hours or frozen. Freeze the burgers individually, separating each with cling film or baking parchment.*

Chicken and pasta with creamy sauce

This delicious dish is likely to be popular. Pouring cream with a fat content of around 10 per cent provides a creamy feel without adding too much saturated fat. The cornflour stabilizes the sauce so it can be frozen.

 5 mins   12–15 mins   4–6 baby portions or 1 adult and 3 baby portions

ingredients

2 tsp **olive oil**
2 **chicken mini-breast fillets,** or 1 small 100g (3½oz) skinless **chicken breast**, diced
1 small **garlic clove**, crushed
45g (1½oz) **button mushrooms**, wiped and sliced
1 tsp **cornflour**
100ml (3½fl oz) **pouring** or **half cream**

50ml (1¾fl oz) **whole milk**
50g (1¾oz) **frozen peas**, cooked
2 tsp chopped **parsley**

Pasta:
For each baby portion, use 15–20g (½–¾oz) dry weight **pasta**, such as pasta bows, penne, or children's pasta shapes

method

1 Boil the pasta in water according to packet instructions, then drain.

2 Meanwhile, heat the oil in a small non-stick saucepan; fry the chicken over a medium heat for 2–3 minutes, stirring frequently.

3 Add the garlic and mushrooms; cook for 5 minutes, or until the chicken is no longer pink inside.

4 Place the cornflour in a small bowl and stir in the cream and milk, then add to the pan, along with the peas and parsley.

5 Bring to a simmering point, stirring continuously. When the sauce thickens, remove from the heat, and cool slightly.

6 Remove a portion for your baby and serve with the cooked pasta.

✳ **Refrigerate** *for up to 24 hours or freeze on the day of cooking in individual pots when cooled.*

Turkey and red pepper patties

Turkey is a great source of vitamin B3, and peppers provide vitamins A and C, making this a nutritious finger food. It can be mashed for babies who prefer to be spoon fed.

 5 mins 14–17 mins 8 little patties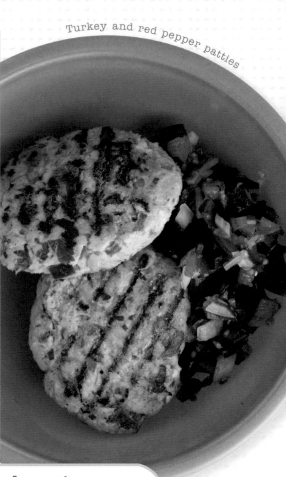

Turkey and red pepper patties

ingredients

1 tbsp **vegetable oil**, plus extra for frying
1 small **onion**, finely chopped
½ large **red pepper**, finely chopped
200g (7oz) **turkey mince**
1 tbsp chopped **parsley**
flour (optional)

method

1 Heat the oil in a non-stick frying pan and fry the onion and red pepper for 4–5 minutes, or until softened.

2 Remove from the heat and cool a little before pulsing to combine with the mince and parsley.

3 On a clean chopping board, form 8 little patties; add flour if too sticky.

4 Heat 1–2 tablespoons of vegetable oil in a non-stick frying pan, and gently fry the patties for 10–12 minutes, or until golden brown, turning over to fry on the other side. Remove from the heat, cool a little, and serve.

✱ **Serve** *with Home-made tomato salsa (see p182) or Peach chutney (see p182).*

✱ **Refrigerate** *in an airtight container for up to 24 hours or freeze when cooled.*

✱ **Variations:** *Use chicken or pork mince instead of turkey. You can add garlic or herbs, such as tarragon, in step 2.*

Bulghur wheat with lamb and aubergine

Bulghur wheat is made by cracking the grains of either whole or husked wheat. Both provide protein and iron as well as dietary fibre. It's ideal for use in one-pot dishes where you can easily add it to stewed meat or vegetables.

 5 mins 20–25 mins 4–6 baby portions

ingredients

200g (7oz) **lean lamb mince**
150g (5½oz) **aubergine**, finely diced
1 small **onion**, finely chopped
1 **garlic clove**, crushed
100g (3½oz) **bulghur wheat**
zest of half a **lemon**, finely grated
1 tbsp **tomato purée**
1 tbsp chopped **parsley**

method

1 Place the lamb and aubergine in a saucepan, and cook over a medium heat for 5 minutes, breaking up the mince with a wooden spoon.

2 When the mince is lightly browned, stir in the onion and garlic, and cook for another 5 minutes, stirring frequently.

3 Add the wheat, lemon zest, tomato purée, and 350ml (12fl oz) water, and bring to a simmering point. Stir, cover, and simmer for 10–15 minutes, or until the water has been absorbed and the wheat is tender.

4 Remove from the heat, stir in the parsley, and allow to cool a little before serving.

✱ **Serve** *with a green vegetable, such as spinach or broccoli.*

✱ **Refrigerate** *for up to 48 hours or freeze on the day of cooking when cooled.*

✱ **Variations:** *You can use beef mince instead of lamb. Add ½ teaspoon of cinnamon for a more Moroccan taste.*

Shepherd's pie

Shepherd's pie (made with lamb) or cottage, pie (made with beef) makes an inexpensive nutritious meal. Rich in easily absorbed iron, this recipe is lovely for babies, toddlers, and adults. Make sure you use lean mince.

 15 mins   35–40 mins   2–3 baby and 3 adult portions

ingredients

vegetable oil, for frying
1 medium **onion**, finely chopped
1 small **leek**, finely chopped
500g (1lb 2oz) extra lean **lamb** or **beef mince**
3 medium **carrots**, peeled and diced
300ml (10fl oz) **water** or diluted **beef stock**
2 **bay leaves**

1 tbsp **cornflour** or **flour**

For the topping:
700g (1¾lb) **floury potatoes**, such as King Edwards, peeled and halved
50ml (1¾fl oz) **semi-skimmed milk**
2 tsp **olive oil spread** or **butter**
black pepper

method

1 Preheat the oven to 200°C (400°F/Gas 6). Heat the oil in a large non-stick saucepan and add the onion, leek, and mince. Fry gently, stirring to break up the mince with a wooden spoon.

2 Add the carrots. Fry until the mince browns and the onion softens. Add the water or stock and bay leaves, then simmer. Cover, reduce the heat, and cook for 15–20 minutes, stirring a little.

3 Boil or steam the potatoes until tender. Drain and mash with the milk, olive oil spread or butter, and pepper. Mix the cornflour with 2 tablespoons of cold water; add to the meat to thicken. Pour into an ovenproof dish, and remove the bay leaves.

5 Spoon or pipe the potato; bake for 20–25 minutes, or until the mixture is piping hot and the potato starting to brown. Remove your baby's portion and cool a little before serving.

✳ Serve *with steamed broccoli, kale or cabbage.*

✳ Cover *and refrigerate for 24 hours or freeze on the day of cooking.*

Beef meatballs in tomato sauce

Meatballs are a family favourite. Whether your baby likes to use her fingers, or to eat mashed meatballs from a spoon, you'll be providing her with an iron-rich meal.

 15 mins   25–30 mins   7–10 baby portions

ingredients

For the sauce:
1 tbsp **vegetable oil**
1 small **onion**, peeled and finely chopped
1 **garlic clove**, crushed
250g (9oz) smooth **passata**
25g (scant 1oz) **sundried tomatoes** in oil, drained and roughly chopped
1 tsp finely chopped **thyme** or **oregano**,

For the meatballs:
250g (9oz) **lean beef mince**
1 slice **wholemeal bread**
½ small **onion**, roughly chopped
few large **basil leaves**
flour (optional)
vegetable oil, for frying

method

1 For the sauce, heat the oil in a non-stick saucepan and gently fry the onion and garlic for 4–5 minutes, or until softened.

2 Add the passata, sundried tomatoes, and thyme or oregano, and bring to a simmering point. Stir, cover, and simmer for 15 minutes, stirring occasionally.

3 For the meatballs, blend the mince, bread, onion, and basil until mixed. Form into 20 small balls, using flour if sticky.

4 Heat 1–2 tablespoons of oil in a non-stick frying pan and fry the meatballs until browned, turning as they cook.

5 Drain on kitchen paper. For each portion, serve 2–3 balls with 1 tablespoon of sauce.

✳ Serve *with rice, mashed potatoes or pasta.*

✳ Refrigerate *for up to 24 hours or freeze in individual portions on day of cooking when cooled.*

✳ Variations: *Use any meat or poultry mince.*

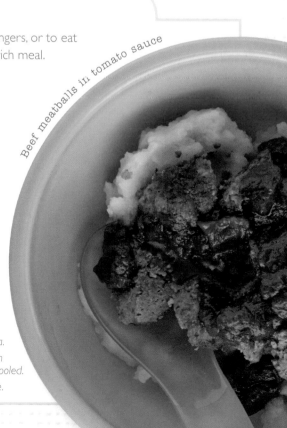

Beef meatballs in tomato sauce

Crispy salmon fingers

Home-made fish fingers are quick to make, and using salmon provides your baby with important omega 3 fatty acids for brain and eye development. These are also ideal for babies who like to feed themselves as they can be held and dipped.

 5–10 mins  12–15 mins   6–8 fingers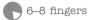

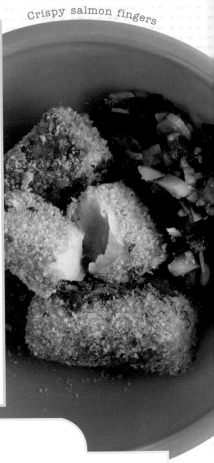

Crispy salmon fingers

ingredients

1 slice day-old, half-and-half **bread** (50 per cent wholemeal), crusts removed
1 tsp finely chopped **parsley**
finely grated **zest of ½ lemon**
1 **egg**
100g (3½oz) skinless **salmon fillet**

method

1 Preheat the oven to 190°C (375°F/Gas 5). Line a baking sheet with non-stick paper or baking parchment.

2 Blend the bread into fine breadcrumbs. Pulse as you add the parsley and lemon zest. Pour the breadcrumb mix into a shallow bowl.

3 Meanwhile, beat the egg in a shallow bowl.

4 Check the fish for bones by running your finger over the surface; remove any you find.

5 Cut into 6 or 8 small pieces. Carefully place one piece in the egg and coat it all over. Using tongs, transfer it to the bowl of breadcrumbs and coat both sides with crumbs. Place the coated piece on the baking sheet and repeat with all the fish.

6 Bake for 6 minutes, then turn over to the other side, and bake until crispy. Allow to cool before serving.

∗ Serve with Avocado dip (see p105), Home-made tomato salsa (see p182), and tomato slices.

∗ The fingers are a little fragile, but can be carefully frozen if separated by greaseproof paper.

∗ Variations: Any firm fish can be used for this, but oily fish contains more omega 3.

Salmon and dill risotto

Babies love rice, and whether they are spoon-fed, or like to get their hands sticky, this risotto provides great nutrition. Ready-chopped frozen spinach is easy to stir in at the end of cooking, saving you time.

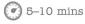 5–10 mins   35–40 mins   3–4 baby or 2 baby and 2 adult portions

ingredients

100g (3½oz) **salmon fillet**
juice of ½ **lemon**
1 tbsp **vegetable oil**
10cm (4in) piece white part of a **leek**, finely chopped
75g (2½oz) **risotto rice**
350–400ml (12–14fl oz) low-salt **vegetable** or **fish stock**
1 tsp **freshly chopped dill**
60g (2oz) frozen chopped **spinach**, defrosted and drained
30g (1oz) **mascarpone** or **cream cheese**
black pepper and **salt**, to serve (optional)

method

1 Preheat the oven to 190°C (375°F/Gas 5).

2 Check the fish for bones by running your finger over the surface, and removing any you find. Place in an ovenproof dish and pour over the lemon juice. Steam, microwave, or bake for 12–15 minutes, or until the fish flakes easily. When cooked, remove the skin and keep warm.

3 Heat the oil in a saucepan and fry the leek for 3–4 minutes, or until soft but not brown.

4 Add the risotto rice and stir in about ⅓ of the stock. Stir and continue cooking over a medium heat, stirring in more liquid until all the fluid has been absorbed.

5 After 30–35 minutes, or when the rice is tender and all the liquid absorbed, stir in the dill and spinach and heat through briefly. Remove from the heat and stir in the mascarpone or cream cheese. Flake the salmon into the risotto and stir to combine.

6 Remove your baby's portion and serve. Season your portion with the pepper and salt, if desired.

∗ Serve with halved cherry tomatoes, steamed cauliflower or carrots.

∗ Freeze on the day of cooking when cooled.

Simple fish pie

Full of calcium, magnesium, and B vitamins, this potato-topped fish pie is a popular family dish. It freezes well, so you can double the mixture and freeze half in a foil tray for days when you have less time to cook.

 20 mins  40–45 mins   2–3 baby and 3 adult portions

ingredients

500g (1lb 2oz) skinless
   white fish fillets
450ml (15fl oz) **whole milk**
2 **bay leaves**
strip of **lemon zest**
vegetable oil, for greasing
20g (¾oz) **butter** or
   monounsaturated spread
30g (1oz) **plain flour**
50ml (1¾fl oz) **half-fat single** or
   pouring **cream**
100g (3½oz) **frozen peas**, thawed
1 tbsp **freshly chopped parsley**

For the topping:

700g (1lb 9oz) **floury potatoes**,
   peeled and quartered
2 tbsp **whole milk**
knob of **butter** or
   monounsaturated spread

method

1 Preheat the oven to 180°C (350°F/Gas 4). Run your finger over the fish fillet to check for bones, removing any you find.

2 Pour the milk into a shallow saucepan or frying pan and add the bay leaves, lemon zest, and fish. Cover and heat very gently to poach the fish.

3 Meanwhile, steam or boil the potatoes until tender. Mash with the milk and spread or butter.

4 When the fish flakes easily, carefully remove from the pan. Oil a shallow ovenproof dish and spread the fish over the base. Remove the lemon zest and bay leaves, and strain the milk into a jug for use in the sauce.

5 To make the sauce, heat the butter or spread in a saucepan and stir in the flour. Cook for 30 seconds, then add the reserved milk, little by little, stirring constantly, until the sauce has thickened. Add the cream, peas, and parsley, and pour over the fish.

6 Spoon or pipe the mashed potatoes over the fish. Bake for 25–30 minutes, or until golden brown. Remove your baby's portion and allow to cool a little before serving.

✳ **Serve** *with more peas, broccoli, and a few carrots.*

✳ **Cover** *with cling film and refrigerate for 24 hours. Alternatively, freeze before baking, and when defrosted (best in the fridge overnight), bake as in step 6, allowing a little longer to ensure it is piping hot.*

Bulghur wheat with currants and chickpeas

Bulghur, bulgur or bulgar wheat makes a moist dish with succulent currants and chickpeas. This is a meal in itself, although it can be served as an accompaniment to a casserole or grilled meat or poultry for older children and adults.

 5–10 mins  25 mins   2 baby and 2–3 adult portions

ingredients

1 tbsp **vegetable oil**
1 medium **onion**,
   finely chopped
150g (5½oz) **butternut
   squash**, finely diced
25g (scant 1oz) **currants**
100g (3½oz) **bulghur wheat**
400g (14oz) can **chickpeas**
   in water, rinsed and
   drained
2 **bay leaves**
1 heaped tbsp chopped
   parsley

method

1 Heat the oil in a large saucepan and gently fry the onion for 5 minutes, or until just softening. Add the butternut squash and continue cooking over a medium heat, stirring frequently for 5 minutes.

2 Stir in the currants, wheat, chickpeas, 500ml (16fl oz) water, and bay leaves, and bring to the boil. Cover, reduce the heat, and simmer for 15 minutes. In the last few minutes of cooking, remove the bay leaves, and stir in the parsley.

3 When the wheat is tender, remove from the heat, and allow to stand for 5 minutes. Remove your baby's portion and allow to cool a little before serving. You can also mash, if required, to an appropriate consistency for your baby before serving.

✳ **Serve** *with steamed green beans, broccoli or halved cherry tomatoes.*

✳ **Refrigerate** *for up to 24 hours.*

✳ **Variations:** *Use raisins instead of currants. Chickpeas can also be replaced with any type of cooked beans.*

Cowboy beans with cornmeal topping

Cornmeal or fine polenta makes a lovely crust on top of spicy beans. Beans supply a host of different B vitamins, as well as some iron, and the vitamin C in the tomato sauce helps the iron to be absorbed.

 10 mins   35–40 mins   4 baby and 2 adult portions   ❄

ingredients

1 tbsp **vegetable oil**, plus extra for greasing
1 small **onion**, finely chopped
75g (2½oz) **mushrooms**, halved and sliced
250g (9oz) cooked or canned **beans** of your choice, such as pinto, **cannellini**, or **borlotti**
400g (14oz) can chopped **tomatoes** in juice
2 tbsp **tomato purée**
1 tbsp chopped **thyme**

For the topping:
2 large **eggs**
50g (1¾oz) fine **cornmeal** or **polenta**
50g (1¾oz) **plain flour**
1 tsp **baking powder**
black pepper
50g (1¾oz) **hard cheese**, such as Cheddar, grated (optional)

method

1 Preheat the oven to 190°C (375°F/ Gas 5) and grease a medium-sized ovenproof dish.

2 For the beans, heat the oil in a non-stick saucepan and gently fry the onion for 5 minutes, or until softened, stirring frequently. Add the mushrooms and continue to cook for 3–4 minutes, or until the mushrooms soften.

3 Add the beans, tomatoes, purée, 100ml (3½fl oz) water, and thyme. Bring to the boil, and pour into the dish.

4 For the topping, beat the eggs well with 50ml (1¾fl oz) water and stir in the dry ingredients. Add the grated cheese, if using.

5 Pour the topping mix over the beans. Bake for 25–30 minutes, or until the topping is risen and firm. Remove your baby's portion and mash, if required. Allow to cool a little, and serve. Season your portion to taste.

✳ **Serve** *with a spoon of reduced-fat soured cream and steamed spinach.*
✳ **Refrigerate** *for 24 hours. The cooked bean mixture can be frozen when cooled separately or as a whole dish.*
✳ **Variations:** *For your portion, you can add chilli sauce or smoky chipotle paste.*

Creamy avocado pasta

This easy sauce can be made while the pasta cooks. Serve alongside the pasta for dipping, or chop or mash the sauce and pasta to a suitable texture for your baby.

 5 mins   12–15 mins   1 baby and 1 adult portion

ingredients

90g (3¼oz) **penne pasta**
1 ripe **avocado**, halved and stone removed
2 tbsp **olive oil**
3–4 **basil leaves**, washed

grated **zest** of ½ **lemon**
2 tsp **lemon juice**
50g (1¾oz) **Parmesan cheese**, grated

method

1 Boil the pasta in water according to the packet instructions.

2 Meanwhile, scoop out the avocado flesh using a spoon and process with all the other ingredients until smooth.

3 When the pasta is cooked, drain, and remove 20–30g (¾–1oz), or 1 tablespoon, for your baby's portion. Season your portion to taste and enjoy!

✳ **Serve** *with a few halved cherry tomatoes or some steamed broccoli.*
✳ *Not suitable for storage.*

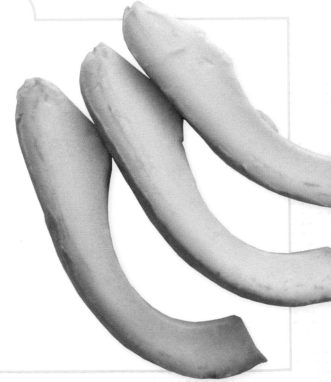

Fruity couscous with peanut sauce

Dried fruit, whether raisins, dried prunes, apricots or currants all provide iron. This can be served as a family side dish without the peanut sauce, but the peanuts provide protein, healthier fats, and iron, zinc, and copper.

 10 mins   10 mins   2 baby and 2 adult portions

ingredients

150g (5½oz) **couscous**
50g (1¾oz) **currants**, or any dried fruit of your choice, finely chopped
150g (5½oz) **peas**, cooked
For the peanut sauce:
25g (scant 1oz) **creamed coconut**
100g (3½oz) **crunchy peanut butter**, preferably salt- and sugar-free or reduced
1 **garlic clove**, crushed (optional)

method

1 Place the couscous and currants in a large bowl and pour over 350ml (12fl oz) boiling water. Leave to stand until the water is all absorbed.

2 Meanwhile, place all the ingredients for the peanut sauce together with 150ml (5fl oz) hot water in a small saucepan, and gently heat, stirring continuously, until the sauce is smooth and well combined.

3 Stir the cooked peas into the couscous. Serve a portion of the couscous mixture topped with the peanut sauce.

✱ **Serve** *with a few halved cherry tomatoes. If your baby prefers, serve the peanut sauce separately with Flaked fish (p106) or Mini lamb and mint balls (p109).*

✱ **Refrigerate** *separately in airtight containers for 24 hours.*

✱ **Variations:** *Add sweetcorn instead of peas. For an adult sauce, add 1 tablespoon of soy sauce, 2 teaspoons of fish sauce, and 1 tablespoon of chopped coriander when your baby has had his serving.*

Vegetarian shepherd's pie

This potato-topped lentil and vegetable dish is a great source of plant based iron. If you are bringing up your baby as a vegetarian, then don't forget to give him a well-diluted drink of unsweetened fruit juice with his main meals.

 15–20 mins   60 mins   8 baby or 2 baby and 2–3 adult portions

ingredients

vegetable oil, for greasing
150g (5½oz) whole **lentils**
1 **bay leaf**
2 tbsp **olive oil**
1 medium **onion**, finely chopped
1 medium **aubergine**, cut into 1cm (½in) cubes
100g (3½oz) **mushrooms**, roughly chopped
1 tbsp freshly chopped, or 1 tsp dried, **marjoram**
1 tsp **mushroom ketchup** (optional)
750g (1lb 10oz) **floury potatoes**
2 tbsp **whole milk**
10g (¼oz) **butter** or **olive spread**

method

1 Preheat the oven to 200°C (400°F/Gas 6). Grease a 2-litre (3½-pint) ovenproof dish.

2 Rinse the lentils in a sieve, place with the bay leaf in a saucepan with cold water, and bring to the boil, simmering until softened. Timing varies with different lentils, so check the instructions. Drain, removing the bay leaf, and reserve some of the cooking liquid.

3 Heat the olive oil in a large non-stick saucepan and fry the onion for 4–5 minutes, or until it starts to soften. Stir in the aubergine and mushrooms, and cook over a low heat for 10 minutes, stirring occasionally, and adding a little water, if necessary, to prevent sticking.

4 Add the marjoram, mushroom ketchup, if using, the cooked and drained lentils, and

200ml (7fl oz) of the reserved cooking liquid, with additional water, if required. Bring to a simmer, stir, and cook for 10 minutes, or until all the ingredients are fully softened.

5 If the vegetables look large for your baby, pulse half the mixture lightly and combine with the remaining mixture.

6 Meanwhile, peel, quarter, and boil the potatoes until tender. Drain and mash with the milk and butter. Pour the lentil mixture into the dish, and spread the mashed potato on top.

7 Bake for 25 minutes, or until the top is lightly browned and the mixture piping hot. Cool a little before serving your baby.

✱ **Serve** *with steamed green beans, or broccoli florets or cauliflower.*

✱ **Refrigerate** *for up to 48 hours or freeze on the day of cooking when cooled.*

✱ **Variations:** *If you don't have time to cook lentils, buy pouches or cans of cooked unsalted lentils. If you eat fish, use 1 teaspoon of Worcestershire sauce instead of mushroom ketchup.*

Baked stuffed apple

In the UK, Bramley cooking apples are traditionally used for this recipe, as their flesh becomes fluffy and meltingly soft. However, you can use eating apples as well, just choose a sharp variety.

 5 mins   45 mins   2 baby and 1 adult portion

ingredients

2 small **Bramley apples**
or 2 regular **eating apples**
2–3 tbsp **mincemeat**
10g (¼oz) **butter**

method

1 Preheat the oven to 170°C (325°F/Gas 3).

2 Wash the apples and remove the core. Score around the circumference of each apple to prevent it from splitting while cooking.

3 Place the apples in a small ovenproof dish and fill with the mincemeat, pushing in as much as you can. Place a knob of butter on top of each, and bake until the apples are really tender, about 45 minutes.

4 Cool to just above room temperature. To serve, scoop out some of the soft flesh and filling, and place in a bowl. Mash if required.

✻ **Serve** *with vanilla ice cream or 1 spoon of plain yogurt.*

✻ **Refrigerate** *in an airtight container for 24 hours.*

✻ **Variations:** *Instead of mincemeat, use 25g (scant 1oz) chopped dried fruit, such as raisins, prunes or apricots, mixed with 2 teaspoons of dark brown sugar or maple syrup and a pinch of mixed spice.*

Baked spiced peach

Stone fruits such as peaches, nectarines, and plums make a deliciously simple dessert with minimum effort. Though baked, the peaches still provide plenty of vitamin C.

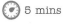 5 mins   15–20 mins   2 baby portions

ingredients

1 tsp unsalted **butter**,
plus extra for greasing
1 large **peach** or
nectarine

1 tsp **demerara sugar**
whole **nutmeg**, to grate

method

1 Preheat the oven to 200°C (400°F/Gas 6). Lightly grease a small ovenproof dish.

2 Peel the peach by pulling off the skin if it comes off easily, or dipping in boiling water for 20 seconds, and then removing. Halve the peach, remove the stone, and cut each half into 4–5 slices. Place in the dish.

3 Sprinkle over the sugar and place the butter on top. Grate nutmeg lightly over the fruit and bake for 15–20 minutes, or until the fruit is tender.

4 Cool and offer half the slices to your baby, storing the other half for another meal.

✻ *Your baby may enjoy dipping these in plain yogurt.*

✻ **Refrigerate**, *covered in cling film, for 24 hours.*

✻ **Variations:** *Plums or apricots can also be used instead of peaches, with the stones removed.*

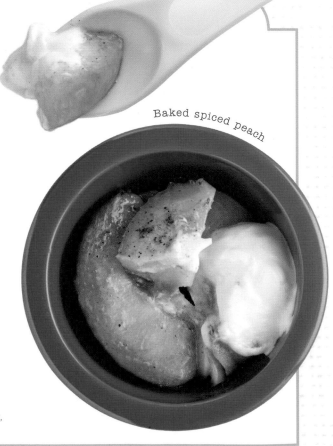

Baked spiced peach

Stewed summer berries

This easy fruit compote is a rich source of vitamin C. Purple and red fruits are an excellent way to eat the protective plant substances polyphenols, which boost your baby's immune system.

 5 mins   5 mins   4–6 baby portions

ingredients

200g (7oz) pack frozen mixed **summer fruit**, thawed, or an equivalent of fresh summer berries and currants, such as:
100g (3½oz) **strawberries**
50g (1¾oz) **blackcurrants** or **blueberries**
50g (1¾oz) **raspberries**
50ml (1½fl oz) unsweetened **apple** or **red grape juice**

method

1 If using fresh fruit, wipe with damp kitchen paper to remove any dust. Remove any stalks from the strawberries and halve or quarter, if large.

2 Place all the fruits in a small saucepan and add the apple or red grape juice.

3 Bring very gradually to a simmering point, and remove from the heat.

4 Allow to cool, and serve at room temperature.

✳ **Serve** *with 1 spoon of Greek yogurt or fromage frais.*
✳ **Refrigerate** *in an airtight container for 2–3 days or freeze when cooled.*

Exotic fruit salad

Fresh fruit provides an abundance of vitamin C and "phytonutrients": plant substances that boost health. Either cut up the fruit into larger pieces for your baby to hold, or chop up finely for spoon feeding. The fruit can be prepared and refrigerated for 24 hours, but add the banana just before serving.

 10 mins   3–4 baby portions

ingredients

1 **kiwi fruit**, peeled and halved
2–3 slices of **mango**
1 small slice **cantaloupe melon**

2–3 tbsp unsweetened **pineapple juice**
few slices of ½ small **banana**

method

1 Cut the kiwi fruit either into slices or chop finely and place in a bowl.

2 Cut the mango and melon into cubes, the size depending on your baby's needs, and add to the bowl.

3 Pour over the juice, stir in the banana, and serve at once.

✳ **Serve** *with 1 spoon of yogurt or vanilla ice cream.*
✳ **Refrigerate** *in an airtight container for 24 hours.*
✳ **Variations:** *Add papaya or pineapple cubes.*

Passion fruit and mango dessert

This is an idyllic combo. Although pricey, passion fruit makes a lovely addition to this creamy dessert. You can strain out the pips, or leave them in for an older child.

 5 mins   2 baby portions

ingredients

½ ripe **passion fruit**
2 tbsp **mango purée**

30g (1oz) or 1 heaped tbsp **mascarpone**

method

1 Scrape the seeds from the passion fruit into a small sieve and push through the juice until you are left with seeds in the sieve. Discard the seeds.

2 Pour the juice into a small bowl and mix with the purée.

3 Beat the mascarpone with a wooden spoon until smooth, and carefully mix in the mango and passion fruit mix.

4 Pour into 2 very small plastic bowls, cover, and chill.

✳ **Serve** *with fresh peeled mango pieces.*
✳ **Refrigerate** *in an airtight container for up to 24 hours.*
✳ **Variation:** *If including the passion fruit seeds, omit steps 1 and 2, and once the mango and mascarpone are mixed, squeeze the passion fruit over the top. A little finely grated lime zest provides a nice zing for adults.*

Mandarin jelly

Sweetened only with the fruit and its own juice, mandarin jelly is a nutritious alternative to shop-bought jelly. Even with heat treatment, a can of mandarins provides a good source of vitamin C.

 5 mins   6 baby portions

ingredients

300g (10½oz) can **mandarins** in fruit juice

8g (¼oz) or 1 heaped tsp **gelatin** unsweetened **orange juice**

method

1 Drain the mandarins from the can, reserving the fruit juice, and divide between 6 small dishes or one large one.

2 Place 3 tablespoons of very hot, but not boiling, water in a small bowl and sprinkle over the gelatin. Allow to

stand for 5 minutes, then stir until dissolved.

3 Mix the reserved juice with the gelatin and enough orange juice to make 300ml (10fl oz). Pour into the dish(es) and refrigerate until the jelly is set.

✱ **Refrigerate** *covered in cling film, for up to 48 hours.*

✱ **Variations:** *Try a can of apricots in juice, adding any unsweetened juice of your choice. You can add a little grated fresh orange or lemon zest for a more citrus flavoured tang.*

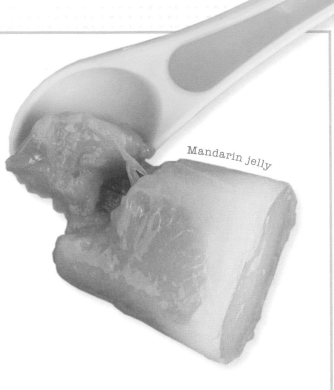

Mandarin jelly

Basic pancake recipe

Using a very hot, well-used, frying or pancake pan that doesn't allow batter to stick is the key to making good pancakes. The right pan means you don't need more than a dribble of oil for each pancake.

 5 mins 10 mins 6 x 20cm(8in) pancakes

ingredients

125g (4½oz) **plain white flour**
1 **egg**
225ml (7½fl oz) **semi-skimmed milk**
1 tbsp **vegetable oil**

✱ **Refrigerate** *for 24 hours or freeze on the day of cooking when cooled.*

method

1 Place the flour, egg, and milk in a blender or processor and combine to make a pouring batter.

2 Meanwhile, heat a pancake or frying pan until hot, and spoon in ½ tsp of oil. Bear in mind that hot oil expands so you won't need as much as you suspect.

3 Swirl the oil around the pan, and pour in a ladleful of batter, swirling this around the hot pan just to coat the base.

4 Fry over a medium–high heat until the batter has just dried, starts to peel away from the sides, and the base is lightly browned. Toss or turn the pancake over and cook for another few seconds.

5 Tip out onto a plate and repeat steps 3 and 4 until all the batter is used up.

6 The pancakes can be interleaved with cling film or greaseproof paper and frozen when cooled, or used fresh.

Pear and raisin oat crumble

Crumbles are a favourite pudding, and the topping can be prepared and refrigerated for a few days, or frozen. The fruit base can be varied according to the season, and you could equally well use plums, apples, gooseberries or a combination of berries with these. Use unsweetened fruit juice to stew the fruit initially and only add sugar if necessary, as the topping contains sugar.

 10 mins   40–45 mins   2 baby and 3 adult portions

ingredients

vegetable oil, for greasing
400–450g (14oz–1lb) or 3 **pears**, peeled, cored, and roughly chopped
50g (1¾oz) **raisins**
½ tsp **ground cinnamon**
50ml (1¾fl oz) unsweetened **apple juice**

For the crumble topping:
100g (3½oz) **plain white flour**
75g (2½oz) **butter** or **unsaturated margarine**
50g (1¾oz) **rolled oats**
100g (3½oz) **demerara sugar**

method

1 Preheat the oven to 190C (375°F/ Gas 5). Lightly grease a 1.5-litre (2¾-pint) ovenproof dish.

2 Place the pears, raisins, cinnamon, and apple juice in a saucepan and gently stew for 5 minutes, or until the pears begin to soften.

3 Meanwhile, sieve the flour into a bowl. Rub in the butter or margarine until the mixture resembles breadcrumbs. Stir in the oats and sugar.

4 Spoon the pear mixture and cooking juices into the dish and sprinkle over the crumble topping. Bake for 30–35 minutes, or until the crumble is crispy and a light golden colour.

5 Remove your baby's portion and ensure that it is not too much above room temperature before serving.

＊Serve *with 1 spoon of Greek yogurt, custard or ice cream.*
＊Refrigerate *for 48 hours or freeze when cooled.*

Apple sponge pudding

Also known as Eve's pudding after naughty Eve who took the apple from the tree of knowledge. And tempting it is, as it is a deliciously simple sponge cake topping with moist apples underneath.

 10 mins   30–35 mins   4 baby and 2 adult portions

ingredients

vegetable oil, for greasing
300g (10 ½ oz) or 1 large **Bramley apple**, or any other cooking apples
25g (scant 1oz) light **muscovado sugar**
grated **zest** of ½ **lemon**

For the sponge:
50g (1¾oz) **butter** or **unsaturated margarine**, softened
50g (1¾oz) **caster sugar**
1 large **egg**
50g (1¾oz) **plain white flour**
25g (scant 1oz) **wholemeal flour**
1 tsp **baking powder**
few drops **vanilla extract**

method

1 Preheat the oven to 190°C (375°F/ Gas 5). Lightly grease a 1.5-litre (2¾-pint) ovenproof dish, preferably tall, not shallow.

2 Peel and core the apple and slice finely. Mix with the muscovado sugar and lemon zest and sprinkle with 1 tablespoon of water. Spoon into the prepared dish and set aside while you make the sponge.

3 Place all the sponge ingredients in a bowl and mix together well with an electric hand-held mixer.

4 Spoon the sponge over the prepared apple mixture. Don't worry if it doesn't close up all the gaps as this will happen when it cooks. Bake for 30–35 minutes, or until the sponge is set and the apple soft when pierced with a knife.

5 Remove your baby's portion and ensure it is not too much above room temperature before serving.

＊Serve *with 1 spoon of Greek yogurt or vanilla ice cream.*
＊Refrigerate *in an airtight container or freeze when cooled.*
＊Variations: *Add a handful of raisins or other dried fruits, chopped, if large, to the apple mixture.*

Bread and butter pudding

A classic British pudding, bread and butter pudding is an economical way of using up day-old bread.
It is also a great way of providing a calcium-rich dessert that makes a change from yogurt or fromage frais.

 5 mins   30–35 mins   2 baby and 1 adult portion

ingredients

vegetable oil, for greasing
4 thin slices **white bread**
15g (½oz) **unsalted butter**
30g (1oz) **raisins**
½ tsp **ground cinnamon**
1 large **egg**
175ml (6fl oz) **whole milk**
10g (¼oz) **caster sugar**
nutmeg, to grate

method

1 Preheat the oven to 180°C (350°F/Gas 4). Lightly grease a shallow 600ml (1 pint) ovenproof dish.

2 Remove the crusts from the bread, butter each slice on one side, and cut into triangles. Arrange a layer of bread at the base of the dish, with the buttered side facing up. Sprinkle in some raisins and cinnamon. Repeat the process, finishing with a layer of bread.

3 Crack the egg into a bowl, then whisk in the milk, and three quarters of the sugar. Pour over the prepared bread layers and grate over some nutmeg. Sprinkle over the remaining sugar and leave to stand for 30 minutes.

4 Place the dish into the oven and bake for 30–35 minutes, or until the custard has set and the top is golden brown.

＊**Serve** with 1 spoon of plain Greek yogurt or a few slices of fresh fruit.

＊**Refrigerate** in an airtight container for 24 hours.

＊**Variations:** Any dried fruit can be used, chopped, if large. You can also use currant or fruit bread, panettone or brioche.

Apricot and almond pudding

This upside-down pudding is a simple cake mix with fruit and ground almonds. Here, ripe apricots are used, or use canned apricots in juice, fresh plums or peaches. Make a large family pudding or individual ones in ramekins.

 10 mins   15–18 mins   3–4 baby and 2 adult portions   ❄

ingredients

vegetable oil, for greasing
2 large ripe **apricots**, halved
   and stoned
30g (1oz) **caster sugar**
30g (1oz) **unsalted butter**

or **monounsaturated spread**
1 **egg**
30g (1oz) **white flour**
1 tsp **baking powder**
15g (½oz) **ground almonds**

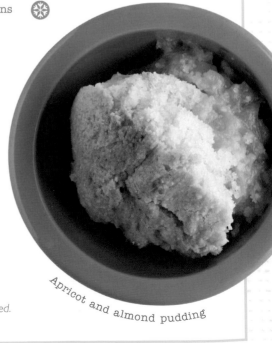

Apricot and almond pudding

method

1 Preheat the oven to 200°C (400°F/ Gas 6). Lightly grease 4 small ramekins or one 12–15cm (5–6in) shallow ovenproof dish.

2 Cut the apricots into slices. Arrange at the base of the ramekins or dish.

3 Beat together the sugar and butter in a small bowl until they are fluffy, and then beat in the egg.

4 Sieve the flour and baking powder and stir into the mixture along with the ground almonds.

5 Spoon the mixture over the apricots and bake for 15–18 minutes, or until the topping is lightly browned and bounces back when gently pressed. Cool, turn it upside down in a small dish, and serve.

＊**Serve** with plain yogurt or a scoop of dairy ice cream.

＊**Refrigerate**, covered with cling film, or freeze on the day of cooking when cooled.

＊**Variations:** Almonds can be replaced with 15g (½oz) of flour.

Blackberry apple cobbler

Fruit puddings do contain sugar and fat, but can be a good way to encourage fruit eating. This cobbler has a sloppy mixture that lets the fruit bubble up through the topping.

 10 mins   35–40 mins 2 baby and 3 adult portions

ingredients

vegetable oil, for greasing
350g (12oz) or 1 large **cooking apple**, peeled, cored, quartered, and sliced
150g (5½oz) **blackberries**, fresh or frozen
3 tbsp unsweetened **apple juice**
1 tbsp **sugar**, if desired

For the topping:
150g (5½oz) **white flour**
75g (2½oz) **wholemeal flour**
2 tsp **baking powder**
50g (1¾oz) **butter** or **unsaturated margarine**
50g (1¾oz) **caster sugar**
grated **zest** of 1 **lemon**
100ml (3½fl oz) **semi-skimmed milk**
1 tbsp **demerara sugar**

method

1 Preheat the oven to 180°C (350°F/Gas 4). Lightly grease a 1.5-litre (2¼-pint) ovenproof dish.

2 Place the apple, blackberries, and apple juice in a saucepan and simmer for 5 minutes to begin to soften the fruit. Taste, and add sugar only if necessary. Transfer to the ovenproof dish.

3 Meanwhile, sieve together the flours and baking powder into a bowl, adding any remaining bran that remains in the sieve.

4 Rub in the butter or margarine until it looks like breadcrumbs. Add the caster sugar, lemon zest, and mix in the milk to make a sticky mixture. Using 2 teaspoons, drop scoops of the mixture over the fruit, and sprinkle with the demerara sugar.

5 Bake for 30–35 minutes, or until the scone mixture is cooked through and looks golden brown. Remove your baby's portion and ensure it is not too much above room temperature before serving.

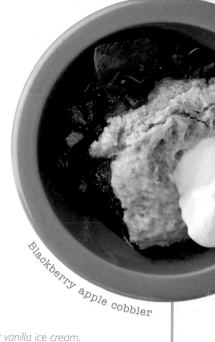

Blackberry apple cobbler

✱ *Serve with 1 spoon of Greek yogurt, crème fraîche or vanilla ice cream.*

✱ *Refrigerate for up to 48 hours or freeze on the day of cooking when cooled.*

✱ *Variations: Try with apple, blackcurrants or redcurrants, berries of all types, or stone fruits. Sweeten only if necessary.*

Baked egg custard

This traditional nursery food is high in protein and calcium, and easy to eat. Rather than cooked in a pastry case, these are baked in small ramekins that can be stored for 24 hours in the fridge.

 5 mins   15–20 mins 3 baby portions

ingredients

vegetable oil, for greasing
1 **egg**
¼ tsp **vanilla extract**
2 tsp **sugar**
150ml (5fl oz) **whole milk**
nutmeg, to grate

method

1 Preheat the oven to 190°C (375°F/Gas 5). Grease 3 small ramekins or ovenproof dishes.

2 Beat the egg well in a bowl with the vanilla extract and sugar. Heat the milk until it is hot, but not boiling, and whisk into the egg mixture.

3 Strain the egg custard into the ramekins and grate a little nutmeg over the top.

4 Place the ramekins in an ovenproof dish and fill the dish up to 1–2cm (½–¾in) with water. Carefully transfer to the oven and bake for around 15 minutes or until set, depending on the depth of the custard. Remove from the oven, cool, and serve or chill until required.

✱ **Serve** *with fresh fruits or Stewed summer berries (see p191).*

✱ **Refrigerate** *for up to 24 hours.*

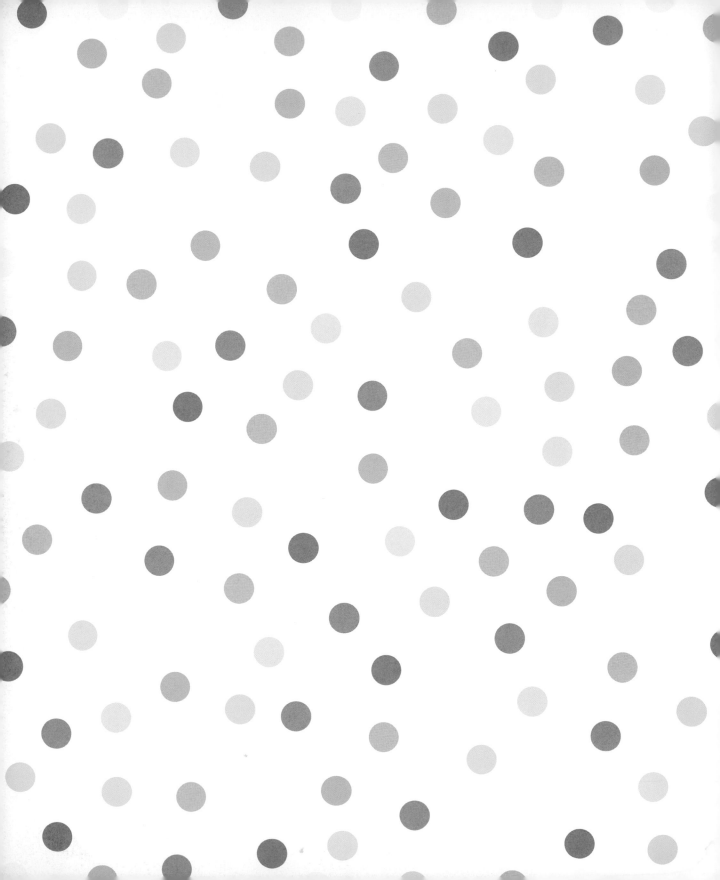

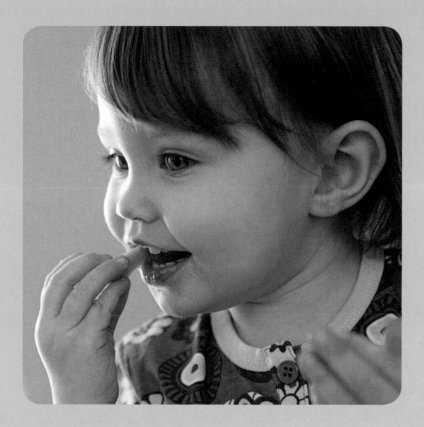

Toddler to *preschool*

Your independent toddler is rapidly developing her own tastes and preferences, which means it's as important as ever now to keep offering healthy foods that provide the range of nutrients she needs to grow and thrive. Continuing the good work of the first months of weaning will help cement healthy eating habits that will stay with your child into adulthood.

Your child's *balanced* diet

You may be breathing a sigh of relief that the early months of feeding are over and your toddler is eating a range of foods, but this is not the time to let up on ensuring she has a nutritious, balanced diet. As your toddler joins in more with family meals, it can be easy to forget that, as with younger babies, toddlers have high nutritional needs. In fact, your toddler uses three times the energy that you do per kilo of body weight. She needs calories not just for growth, but for her increased mobility, too.

Your energetic toddler

Once your child is up on her feet, she'll be burning off plenty of calories as she walks, runs, and starts to explore. This means her need for calories and other important nutrients such as protein, vitamins, and minerals increases. You need to ensure that the foods and drinks she has are nutrient-dense – which means that for every mouthful she receives a good dose of a range of important nutrients. There are various ways to achieve this:

- Offer two nutritious snacks, such as fruit slices, cheese cubes or vegetable sticks with a dip, in addition to three meals a day. Think of snacks as healthy mini-meals, rather than a cup of squash and a biscuit.

- Provide vegetables and nutrient-rich meat, poultry, and fish consistently at mealtimes, even if these are sometimes rejected.

- Continue to use full-fat cheese, yogurt and fromage frais, and milk in cooking up to two years as these provide vitamin A, calcium, and calories.

- Introduce some wholegrain foods, such as wholemeal bread and breakfast cereals, but avoid high-fibre cereals containing bran, which interferes with iron absorption.

- Continue to use rapeseed or olive oil in cooking as these are high in healthier monounsaturated fats.

- If you offer cakes or biscuits, stick to the recommended portion sizes (see pp200–203). These foods are high in energy and saturates and have few other useful nutrients, so ideally make healthier versions yourself.

- The toddler years are also a time when your child starts to assert independence. She may refuse foods she previously liked, as she learns there are less nutritious, but tasty foods available. This can lead to deficiencies in iron, zinc, and vitamins A, D, and C, so it's important not to be put off by this tricky phase and maintain the good eating habits you've already established. With some patience and by keeping mealtimes simple with a positive atmosphere and not giving in to demands, it's possible to get through!

Fast foods

Parents are often worried about whether or not toddlers should have fast foods when eating away from home. For an occasional meal, fast food is not going to harm your child, but don't get into the habit of promising this as a treat or reward, as this undermines all the good work you've being doing at home, and make sure it is a rare, rather than regular, occurrence. The portion sizes provided are often far too big for young children, and a toddler may easily have a full day's salt allowance in one meal, or an excessive amount of saturated fat and calories.

You can, of course, make your own healthier versions of these types of meals at home.

Getting enough vitamins and minerals

Surveys show that many toddlers in the UK don't have sufficient iron and zinc, or vitamins A, C, and D in their diet. A lack of these vital nutrients at this developmental stage can have long-term effects on health and development.

- Inadequate iron in toddlers can cause iron-deficiency anaemia (IDA). A toddler with IDA, which can develop as early as one year, may be pale, tired, and irritable, and, if untreated, may suffer delays in mental and motor development.

- Vitamin D is largely made by the action of sunlight on the skin and isn't found in many foods apart from oily fish. Inadequate vitamin D leads to the bone disease rickets, which can become apparent when toddlers begin to walk as their bones haven't developed properly.

- Zinc and vitamins A and C are all crucial for the development of the immune system, and other important functions.

You can ensure your toddler is getting essential minerals and vitamins by:

- giving vitamin drops that contain vitamins A, C, and D as recommended, unless your child is drinking a toddler milk fortified with these.

- including foods that are a good source of iron and zinc (see pp16–17).

- buying breakfast cereals fortified with iron.

- using fortified toddler foods and/or milk occasionally, especially if your toddler is a fussy eater.

You can help your toddler avoid IDA by:

- ensuring she doesn't drink large quantities of cow's milk, which is low in iron and can displace other foods from the diet. Between one and three years of age, a toddler needs only around 300ml (10fl oz) of milk as a drink per day.

- avoiding weaning late, and especially delaying the introduction of iron-rich foods.

- including good sources of iron such as red meat, fish or poultry in your child's diet.

- avoiding an over-reliance on beans, peas, and lentils or green vegetables to provide iron, as iron is less well absorbed from these types of food.

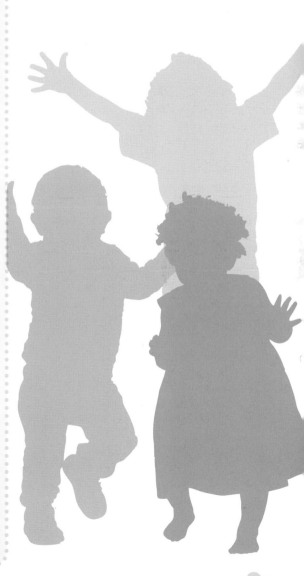

Toddler portions

As your toddler grows, her appetite increases and she'll start to eat larger portions of foods. Parents often worry that their toddler will become overweight if they don't control what they eat. However, research shows that children need to learn to regulate their own appetite and will do this if they are allowed some control. Being over restrictive and controlling won't allow your child to work out when she is full, so offer a range of nutritious foods and let her determine how much of them to eat.

Meeting your child's needs

It's helpful to have some guidance on appropriate portion sizes for different foods to help you get the balance right. The table opposite, based on information from The Infant and Toddler Forum, shows a range of suitable portion sizes for toddlers aged one to four years. Of course, all children have different nutritional needs, and the needs of an 18-month-old toddler will be different to those of a lively three-year-old child.

Toddler drinks

By now your toddler should be using a handled cup rather than a bottle for drinks. Whether with or without a lid will depend on her dexterity.

Cow's milk, which is not recommended under a year due to its low iron content, can be introduced now as a main drink provided your toddler eats well, with plenty of iron-rich foods. If she is a fussy eater, you may want to try one of the growing-up or toddler milks on the market that have added nutrients such as iron, omega 3, and vitamin D.

Continue to give water in preference to cordials, squashes or juice, especially between meals. Apart from contributing to tooth decay, too much juice, or milk, between meals can spoil her appetite. If you wish, unsweetened fruit juices diluted half and half with water at mealtimes will boost her vitamin C intake. Smoothies are best given at mealtimes too as these can fill her up and spoil her appetite: give just 100–150ml (3½–5fl oz).

How much salt?

The table below shows some commonly eaten family foods and the amount of salt per serving they contain. Your toddler needs no more than 2g of salt a day up to the age of three. If she is eating family meals now, continue to avoid adding salt.

FOODS	AMOUNT OF SALT (g)
Cow's milk – full-fat 100ml (3½fl oz)	0.14
1 slice white/wholemeal bread 23g (¾oz)	0.24
Cheddar cheese 30g (1oz) piece	0.5
Plain full-fat yogurt 100g (3½oz)	0.1
Fromage frais, flavoured 100g (3½oz)	0.05
Baked beans, heaped tbsp 50g (1¾oz)	0.35
Tomato ketchup 15g (1 tbsp)	0.4
Bag of potato rings 25g (scant 1oz)	0.6
1 rasher bacon – unsmoked 20g (¾oz)	0.4–0.5
Ham – small slice 10g (¼oz)	0.2
Bag of baked crisps 25g (scant 1oz)	0.3

TYPE OF FOOD	EXAMPLE	RANGE OF PORTION SIZES
BREADS AND SIMILAR FOODS	Bread roll	¼–¾ roll
	Slices of bread/toast	½–1 slice
	Naan bread	⅛–¼ naan
	Chapatti	½–1 chapatti
	Scone – fruit or plain	½–1 small
	Teacake/fruited bun	½–1
	Oatcake	1–2 oatcakes
	Breadsticks	1–3 large breadsticks
	Rice cakes	1–3 medium rice cakes
BREAKFAST CEREALS	Flaked cereals	3–6 tablespoons
	Muesli	2–4 tablespoons
	Wheat biscuits	½–1½ biscuits
	Porridge (made up)	5–8 tablespoons
GRAINS AND PASTA (COOKED)	Couscous	2–4 tablespoons
	Rice	2–5 tablespoons
	Pasta, plain or egg	2–5 tablespoons
	Noodles	½–1 cup
POTATOES	Baked potato	¼–½ medium
	Boiled potato	½–1½ egg-size potato
	Mashed potato	1–4 tablespoons
	Chips	4–8 thick-cut chips
	Roast potato	½–1 potato
VEGETABLES	Broccoli/cauliflower	1–4 small florets
	Cabbage	1–3 tablespoons
	Spinach, kale or spring greens	1–2 tablespoons
	Carrots – cooked	1–3 tablespoons
	Carrot sticks	2–6 sticks
	Celery, cucumber, pepper or other salad vegetables	4–10 sticks or slices
	Tomatoes	¼–1 small tomato
	Cherry tomatoes	1–4 tomatoes
FRUITS	Apple	¼–½ medium apple
	Avocado	½–2 tablespoons
	Banana	½–1 medium banana
	Clementine or similar	½–1 fruit
	Dried apricot/prune	1–4 whole fruit
	Grapes or berries	3–10 small berries
	Kiwi, plum or apricots	½–1 fruit
	Orange	¼–½ orange
	Peach or nectarine	½–1 whole fruit

TYPE OF FOOD	EXAMPLE	RANGE OF PORTION SIZES
FRUITS (continued)	Pear	¼–¾ whole fruit
	Raisins/sultanas	½–1 tablespoon
	Fruit salad	1 small bowl
	Stewed fruit	2–4 tablespoons
MILK AND MILKY PUDDINGS	Full-fat cow's milk	100–120ml (3½–4fl oz)
	Custard	5–7 tablespoons
	Rice pudding/semolina	4–6 tablespoons
YOGURT	Yogurt or calcium-enriched soya dessert	125g (4½oz)
FROMAGE FRAIS	Fromage frais	2 small pots (2 x 60g/2oz)
CHEESE	Grated cheese in sandwich or pizza	2–4 tablespoons
	Cottage or ricotta cheese	½–1 tablespoon
	Processed cheese	1 slice/triangle
MEAT AND POULTRY	Beef or lamb, sliced	½–1 slice
	Pork, chicken or turkey, sliced	1–2 small slices
	Stewed minced meat	2–5 tablespoons
	Lamb's liver	½–1 slice
	Liver pâté	1–2 tablespoons
	Bacon	¼–1 rasher
	Burger	½–1 small burger
	Chicken nuggets	2–4 nuggets
	Sausages	½–1 medium sausage
FISH	Fresh or frozen white or oily	¼–1 small fillet
		1–3 tablespoons
	Canned fish in a sandwich/salad	½ –1½ tablespoons
	Fish fingers	1–2 fingers
	Shellfish – prawns	½–2 tablespoons
EGGS	Poached, fried or boiled	½ to 1 egg
	Scrambled egg	2–4 tablespoons
	Omelette or frittata	Equivalent to 1 egg
NUTS	Ground, chopped or crushed	1–2 tablespoons
	Nut butters	½–1 tablespoon
PULSES (BEANS, LENTILS, AND PEAS)	Baked beans in sauce	2–5 tablespoons
	Chickpeas/ hummus	1–2 tablespoons
	Falafel	1–3 mini falafel (25g/1oz each)
	Dhal/cooked lentils	2–5 tablespoons
	Cooked or canned beans	1–2 tablespoons
CASSEROLES, STEWS, CURRIES, AND STIR FRIES	Meat/fish/chicken/pulses with vegetable sauce and potatoes	3–6 tablespoons

TYPE OF FOOD	EXAMPLE	RANGE OF PORTION SIZES
CASSEROLES, STEWS, CURRIES, AND STIR FRIES (continued)	Meat/fish/chicken/pulses with vegetable sauce. No potatoes	2–5 tablespoons
PASTA DISHES	Lasagne or macaroni cheese	2–5 tablespoons
	Spaghetti bolognaise	3–5 tablespoons
PIZZA	Any topping	1–2 small slices (70g/2½oz)
POTATO-TOPPED PIES	Shepherd's pie	2–5 tablespoons
	Fish pie	2–5 tablespoons
PASTRIES	Quiche or egg flan	½–1½ small slices (30–90g/1–3¼oz)
	Samosa	1–2 small samosas
	Sausage roll	1–3 mini rolls
SOUPS	Vegetable soup	1 small bowl (90–125ml/1¾–4fl oz)
	Soup with meat, fish or pulses	1 small bowl (90–125ml/1¾–4fl oz)
PUDDINGS *	Jelly	2–4 tablespoons
	Ice cream	2–3 heaped tablespoons
	Fruit sorbet	2–4 tablespoons
	Pancake	½–1 small pancake
	Trifle or similar	2–4 tablespoons
	Cake-style pudding, for example apple sponge pudding, or fruit crumble	2–4 tablespoons
CAKES *	Cup cake	½–1 of a 25g/scant 1oz cake
	Muffin	⅛–½ of a 120g/4½oz muffin
	Fruit pie	1 small slice
	Danish pastry/ pain au chocolat	¼–½ medium pastry
	Plain croissant	½–1 croissant; 40g/1½oz
BISCUITS *	Cereal bar	½–1 bar; 20g/¾oz
	Digestive, plain	½–1 biscuit
	Plain (rich tea) or fruit biscuit (garibaldi)	1–2 biscuits
	Cream-filled biscuit	½–1 biscuit
CONFECTIONERY **	Chocolate bar/biscuit	2–4 small square or 1 funsize
	Chocolate buttons	6–8 small buttons
	Popcorn, sweet	1 small cup
CRISPS **	Crisps or savoury puffed shapes	4–6 crisps or shapes
	Tortilla chips	4–6 chips
	French fries – thin from take-away	6–10 fries
	Poppadums	½–1 poppadum

* These foods are high in energy and low in nutrients so observe the serving sizes. Include cakes or biscuits with fruit as a dessert. They can be eaten twice a day in these portion sizes.

** Confectionery and savoury snacks can be offered once or twice a week as part of a meal. Don't use them as rewards, treats or for comfort.

Fussy eaters

Some time in their toddler years, most children decide that foods they previously ate are no longer acceptable. They may also become unwilling to try new foods, a phase called "neophobia", or fear of the new. This is a perfectly normal part of development as children learn to assert their independence, but can be very frustrating for parents who have spent time cooking nutritious meals, only to have them rejected or even thrown on the floor! Fussy eating is often a passing phase, and if your child is growing normally, it is not worth getting overly stressed. That may be easier said than done, but if you show your toddler it is upsetting you, it may be counterproductive, so try to stay calm, and keep offering nutritious meals and snacks.

What can you do?

There are plenty of tactics to try to combat fussy eating:

- Keep an eye on what your child is eating or drinking between meals. Sometimes toddlers drink too much milk between meals, which can spoil their appetite.

- Sit and eat the same meal as your toddler; it is always nicer to eat alongside someone. Don't forget that you are your child's role model, so watching you eat can positively influence her.

- Be positive and calm. Offer your child food, and if it is not eaten just take it away without comment after 15 or so minutes.

- Don't resort to bribes or persuasion. This can reinforce negative messages for your child. "You can have pudding if you eat your meat and vegetables" makes sweet pudding seem like a much more attractive option than nasty vegetables.

- Don't insist your child eats. If she is hungry she will eat, so make sure you offer nutritious food at mealtimes and for snacks, and don't let her fill up on milk and other foods between meals.

- Don't worry if your child goes through a phase of wanting only familiar foods. Continue to offer a range of foods, including the familiar food, and simply take food away when it's left uneaten. Toddlers like familiarity, especially if there has been a change to routine, such as a new sibling, a move, or a new nursery, and a familiar food may help to settle them. This phase will normally pass quite quickly.

- If you're really struggling with mealtimes, ask your partner, relative or a friend to take over occasionally. It may help to diffuse the tension you are feeling.

- Don't become over stressed about small issues. Some children don't like foods to touch one another or be covered with sauce or gravy – they like to see what they are eating. If this isn't too difficult just go with the flow, but if it becomes an issue, do talk to a health professional about it.

> *If your child rejects foods, try not to get too disheartened; continue to offer nutritious foods daily.*

Small is beautiful

If your toddler seems overwhelmed when presented with a big bowl full of food, keep on offering small selections of food, as shown below, which she may find easier to cope with. If she manages to eat the smaller portion, you can always offer her more. Pages 200–203 list the average portion sizes for young children.

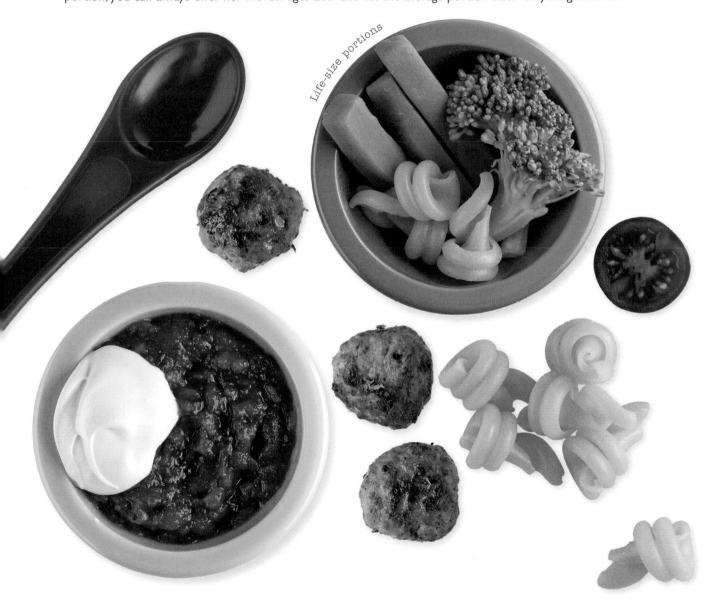

Life-size portions

Family
meal
planner

By now, your little one will be enjoying **family meals** with the rest of the family much of the time. The two sample planners here offer some ideas for nutritious meals to suit the whole family. Snacks are also included as these are an important part of your toddler's diet now. Her little tummy can cope with only small amounts at a time, so to meet her energy needs now that she consumes less milk, she needs to eat smaller, more frequent meals.

Monday

Breakfast
Simple muesli p169 with milk
and slices of banana

Mid-morning snack
Half a buttered currant bun

Lunch
Half small baked potato with
grilled chicken thigh
Healthier coleslaw p211
Fruit yogurt

Mid-afternoon snack
2–3 ready-to-eat apricots

Dinner
Tuna pasta bake p218 with
green beans or broccoli
Stewed apple and
cranberries p129 and custard

Tuesday

Breakfast
Wheat biscuit p70 with
raisins and slices of banana

Mid-morning snack
Apple slices

Lunch
Pea and mint soup p181
with cheese scone p104
Clementine or grapes

Mid-afternoon snack
Breadsticks and cottage
cheese dip p107

Dinner
Mild chilli con carne p217
with rice
Carrot and raisin salad p213
Baked spiced peaches p190
and yogurt

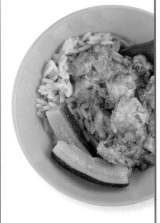

Wednesday

Breakfast
Bircher muesli p98

Mid-morning snack
Fruits of the forest
smoothie p168

Lunch
Scrambled egg p99 on toast
with halved cherry tomatoes
Fromage frais

Mid-afternoon snack
Halved grapes

Dinner
Chicken korma p213 with
rice and cauliflower or peas
Passion fruit and mango
dessert p191

Thursday

Breakfast
Hard-boiled egg with
buttered toast p69
Clementine or peach slices

Mid-morning snack
Half a buttered scone

Lunch
Wholegrain salad p212 with
a spoon of ricotta cheese
Apply plums p129

Mid-afternoon snack
Banana slices

Dinner
Salmon in filo pastry p218
with new potatoes
Sugar snap and apple salad
p210
Chocolate rice pudding p135

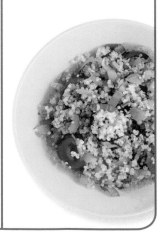

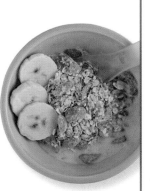

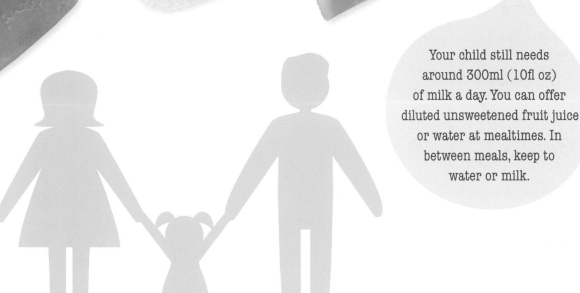

Your child still needs around 300ml (10fl oz) of milk a day. You can offer diluted unsweetened fruit juice or water at mealtimes. In between meals, keep to water or milk.

Friday

Breakfast
Raspberry porridge p99
with berries

Mid-morning snack
Pear or peach slices

Lunch
Tuna and avocado
sandwich p175
with carrot sticks
Banana custard p133

Mid-afternoon snack
Rice cake with peanut butter

Dinner
Moussaka p213
with potatoes,
broccoli or sweetcorn
Fruit fool p133

Saturday

Breakfast
Scrambled egg p99 on toast
with clementine or
strawberry slices

Mid-morning snack
Mixed spice drop scone p99

Lunch
Sweet potato, barley, and
leek soup p102 with fingers
of bread
Stewed summer berries
p191 with yogurt

Mid-afternoon snack
Cubes of cheese

Dinner
Simple fish pie p187 with
peas or sweetcorn
Mandarin jelly p192

Sunday

Breakfast
Spicy banana toast p100
Ready-to-eat apricots or
prunes, halved

Mid-morning snack
Carrot muffin p171

Lunch
Macaroni cheese p125
with halved cherry tomatoes
Mango lolly p132

Mid-afternoon snack
Red pepper sticks with
home-made hummus p111

Dinner
Pork with plums p214
with roast potatoes,
broccoli, and carrots
Chocolate rice pudding p135

Family
meal
planner

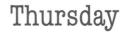

Monday

Breakfast
Hard-boiled egg with
buttered toast p69 and
kiwi slices

Mid-morning snack
Baby breadsticks,
carrots, and
home-made hummus p111

Lunch
Ham and pineapple
pizza p179 with red pepper
and celery fingers
Banana and yogurt

Mid-afternoon snack
Halved grapes

Dinner
Lasagne al forno p217 or
vegetarian lasagne p219 with
cabbage and a bread roll
Apple sponge pudding p193
and custard

Tuesday

Breakfast
Banana bread p168
with butter and
strawberries or blueberries

Mid-morning snack
Mango smoothie p171

Lunch
Pasta, tuna, and
sweetcorn salad p210
with lettuce
Fromage frais

Mid-afternoon snack
Savoury muffin p170

Dinner
Chicken stir fry p214
with noodles
Passion fruit and
mango dessert p191

Wednesday

Breakfast
Simple muesli p169
with chopped ready-to-eat
apricots

Mid-morning snack
Baby blueberry pancake
p169 with butter

Lunch
Hard-boiled egg with
buttered toast p69
Exotic fruit salad p191

Mid-afternoon snack
½ slice toast and cream
cheese p100

Dinner
Salmon in filo pastry p218
with sweet potato
Carrot and raisin salad p213
Lemony ricotta pudding p134

Thursday

Breakfast
Wheat biscuits with
milk p70 and banana slices

Mid-morning snack
Cubes of cheese, half a
buttered English muffin

Lunch
Beetroot and yogurt
salad p208 with ½ slice of
ham and bread and butter
Carrot muffin p171

Mid-afternoon snack
Pitta bread and
peanut butter
Halved cherry tomatoes

Dinner
Cowboy beans with
cornmeal topping p188,
with green beans
or courgettes
Sliced pineapple or mango

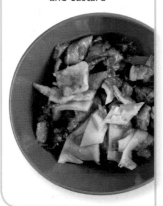

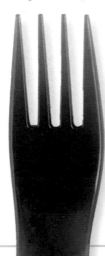

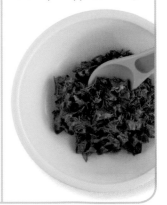

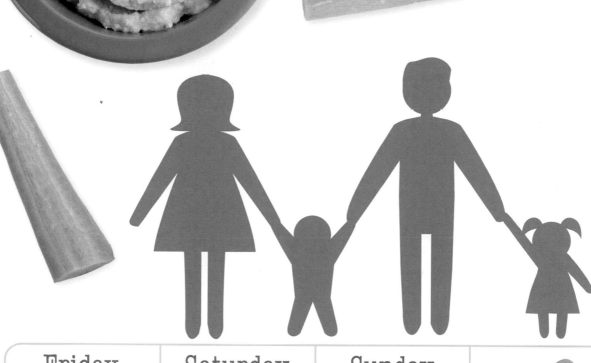

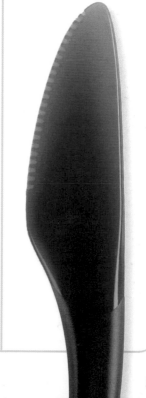

Friday

Breakfast
Mango and vanilla
breakfast p97 with toast and
peanut butter p101

Mid-morning snack
Banana bread p168

Lunch
Sardines on toast p173
with cucumber wedges
Mango or clementines

Mid-afternoon snack
Fruits of the forest
smoothie p168

Dinner
Beef meatballs in tomato
sauce p185 with spaghetti
and lettuce or broccoli
Semolina pudding p134 and
fruit purée pp59–62

Saturday

Breakfast
Sweetcorn and tomato
fritter p172 with halved
cherry tomatoes

Mid-morning snack
Vanilla and banana
smoothie p171

Lunch
Baked potato with spicy
chicken and vegetables p176
Lemony ricotta pudding p134

Mid-afternoon snack
Ready-to-eat prunes
or raisins

Dinner
Pork with plums 214
with rice and cooked
spinach or broccoli
Chocolate rice pudding p135

Sunday

Breakfast
Savoury muffin p170
with fruit yogurt

Mid-morning snack
Avocado dip p105 with
cucumber and pepper

Lunch
Crispy salmon fingers p186,
potato, home-made tomato
salsa p182, peas, and sweetcorn
Fruit fool p133

Mid-afternoon snack
Cheese scone p104 with
cream cheese and tomato slice

Dinner
Turkey and red pepper
patties p184 with peach
chutney p182
Stewed apple and
cranberries p129

Beetroot and yogurt salad

Buy cooked beetroot from the supermarket, or just boil peeled beets and cool, before mixing with a herby tangy yogurt dressing. Beetroot is a great source of the B vitamin folate, as well as being high in potassium.

 5 mins   2 toddler and 2–3 adult portions

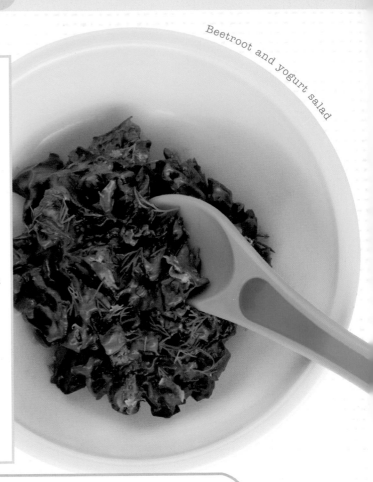

Beetroot and yogurt salad

ingredients

250g (9oz) cooked peeled **beetroot** (not pickled)
3 tbsp **Greek yogurt**

1 tbsp chopped **dill**
1 tbsp chopped **thyme**
juice of ½ **lemon**
grated **zest** of ½ **lemon**

method

1 Slice the beetroot, and then cut each slice into matchstick-sized pieces.

2 Mix the yogurt with the herbs, lemon juice, and the zest, and stir in the beetroot. Serve, or chill until ready to serve.

✱ **Serve** *with grilled chicken or fish.*

✱ **Refrigerate** *for up to 24 hours.*

✱ **Variations:** *Add ¹/₂ small red onion, finely chopped, and I small apple, cored and finely chopped.*

Sugar snap and apple salad

Sugar snaps provide vitamin C in abundance, and the pods are rich in phytonutrients, which protect the body from disease. You can also use mangetout for this salad, which has the same nutritional benefits.

🕐 5–10 mins   🔥 4 mins   ◔ 1–2 toddler and 3 adult portions

ingredients

200g (7oz) **sugar snaps** or **mangetout**
1 large red **eating apple**, washed
50g (1¾oz) **baby spinach** or other salad leaves, washed
1 tbsp toasted **sunflower seeds** (optional)

For the dressing:
1 tbsp **lemon juice**
1 tbsp **olive oil**
1 tsp **runny honey**

method

1 Trim the sugar snaps or mangetout and steam for 3–4 minutes. Dip into cold water to cool, and drain.

2 Make the dressing by whisking all the ingredients together in a bowl.

3 Quarter the apple, remove the core, and cut into small cubes. Stir into the dressing straight away. Cut the sugar snaps into slices around 1cm (½in) in width and mix into the dressing.

4 Arrange the salad leaves on a serving plate, and spoon the mixture over it. Sprinkle over the sunflower seeds, if using, and serve at once.

✱ **Serve** *with a summer barbecue or family dish, such as moussaka (see p215) or lasagne (see p217.*

✱ *Not suitable for storing. Serve within a couple of hours of making.*

Greek-style salads

Colourful and crunchy, Greek salad suggests the essence of summer – Mediterranean warmth, and the sunny flavours of ripe tomatoes and extra virgin olive oil. Keep the salad simple, using just olive oil to dress, and as the feta is salty, don't overdo this. In keeping with the theme, this salad is accompanied by a Greek-style leaf salad.

 5–8 mins   1 toddler and 2 adult portions

ingredients

⅓ **cucumber**, halved lengthwise and thickly sliced
2 large ripe **tomatoes**, cut into chunks
1 small **red onion**, thinly sliced
100g (3½oz) **feta cheese**, cubed
25g (scant 1oz) pitted **black olives**
1 tbsp **olive oil**

For the leaf salad:
8 round (butterhead) **lettuce** leaves
2–3 sprigs of **dill**

For the dressing:
1 tbsp **olive oil**
2 tsp **red wine vinegar**
pinch of **sugar**
black pepper, to taste

method

1 Make the Greek salad by arranging the cucumber, tomatoes, onion, and feta in a salad bowl. Sprinkle over the olives and drizzle with the oil. Cover and set aside while making the other salad.

2 Wash, dry, and gently tear the butterhead leaves and arrange in a salad bowl. Chop the dill and sprinkle this over the lettuce.

3 Make the dressing by combining all the ingredients and pouring over the leaf salad. Serve both salads together.

✱ **Serve** *with wholemeal pitta bread.*
✱ *Not suitable for storing.*

Healthier coleslaw

Shop-bought coleslaw is usually made with fatty mayonnaise, making perfectly healthy vegetables go from low-fat to high-fat. This version uses very low-fat mayonnaise mixed with plain yogurt, which radically cuts the fat content while providing the same taste experience.

 10 mins   2 toddler and 2–3 adult portions

ingredients

2 heaped tbsp low-fat (3 per cent fat or less) **mayonnaise**
2 heaped tbsp **plain yogurt**
200g (7oz) piece **white cabbage**
2 medium **carrots**, peeled
2 sticks **celery**, trimmed and washed

50g (1¾oz) **raisins**, or dried sweetened **cranberries**
1 tbsp **lemon** or **lime juice**
black pepper, to taste (optional)

method

1 Mix the mayonnaise and yogurt in a large bowl. Shred the cabbage very finely and add to the bowl.

2 Coarsely grate the carrots, finely chop the celery, and mix into the bowl.

3 Stir in the raisins or cranberries and lemon juice, and season with the black pepper, if desired. Cover and chill until required.

✱ **Serve** *with baked potatoes, grilled meat or poultry.*
✱ **Refrigerate** *in an airtight container for up to 24 hours.*

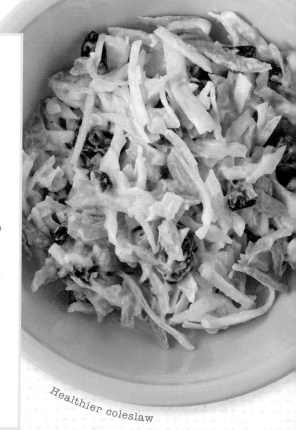

Healthier coleslaw

Wholegrain salad

This colourful vitamin-C rich salad is a great accompaniment to grilled chicken or fish. This version uses quinoa, but it can be made with brown rice, barley, bulghur wheat or wholegrain couscous. Just cook the grain according to the instructions and mix with the other ingredients.

 10 mins　　 10–12 mins　　 2 toddler and 2–3 adult portions

ingredients

120g (4½oz) **quinoa**
200g (7oz) ripe **cherry tomatoes**, quartered
1 medium **yellow** or **orange pepper**, finely diced

1 heaped tbsp **basil leaves**, finely chopped or torn
2 tbsp **extra virgin olive oil**
black pepper, to taste

method

1 Cook the quinoa in unsalted boiling water according to the packet instructions; drain in a sieve, and rinse with cold water to cool.

2 Place the quinoa in a serving bowl and stir in all the remaining ingredients. Serve at once, or cover and chill for use later the same day.

✳ **Serve** *with grilled chicken thighs and Healthier Coleslaw (see p211) for a delicious summer meal.*

✳ **Refrigerate** *and use within 24 hours.*

✳ **Variations:** *Try peppers of different colours. Replace the oil with 50g (1¾oz) drained sundried tomatoes in oil, and 1 tablespoon of the accompanying oil.*

Wholegrain salad

Pasta, tuna, and sweetcorn salad

A family standby, readily eaten by all, this salad has two alternative dressings, one the more traditional creamy tomato, the other a fresher lemony dressing.

 10 mins　　 10–12 mins　　 1–2 toddler and 3 adult portions

ingredients

200g (7oz) **pasta bows** or other shapes
150g (5½oz) **sweetcorn**, canned in water, or frozen
225g (8oz) can **tuna** in water, drained and flaked
4 **spring onions**, trimmed and finely sliced

For dressing 1:
2 tbsp **reduced-fat mayonnaise**

2 tbsp **Greek yogurt**
1 tbsp **tomato purée**
1 tsp **lemon juice**
black pepper, to taste

For dressing 2:
1 tbsp **lime** or **lemon juice**
1 tbsp **olive oil**
½ tsp **caster sugar**
black pepper, to taste

To finish:
1 tbsp chopped **parsley**
2 tbsp **pine nuts**, toasted (optional)

method

1 Cook the pasta in boiling water until just tender, then drain. Rinse in cold water and drain again thoroughly.

2 If using frozen sweetcorn, boil for 2–3 minutes, drain, and cool. Mix the pasta, sweetcorn, and tuna in a large bowl, and add the spring onions.

3 Make either dressing by combining the ingredients in a small bowl and stirring into the pasta salad to coat the ingredients. Sprinkle the parsley and pine nuts, if using, and serve at once, or chill until required.

✳ **Serve** *with tomato salad or a simple leaf salad.*

✳ **Refrigerate** *in an airtight container for up to 24 hours without the pine nuts.*

Carrot and raisin salad

This delicious carrot salad contains juicy segments of orange to boost your baby's vitamin A and C levels. The raisins also provide a sweet contrast that your baby will enjoy.

 10 mins   2 toddler and 3 adult portions

ingredients

300g (10½oz) **carrots**, peeled or scrubbed, trimmed, and finely grated
50g (1¾oz) **raisins**
1 large **orange**
1 tbsp **poppy seeds** (optional)
1 tbsp chopped **parsley**

For the dressing:
1 tbsp **olive oil**
1 tbsp **lime juice**
1 tsp **runny honey**

method

1 In a large bowl, mix together the carrots and raisins. Using a sharp knife, peel the orange. Holding the orange over the bowl to catch any drips, cut away the flesh of each segment, halve, and add to the salad. Stir in the poppy seeds, if using, and parsley.

2 Meanwhile, make the dressing by whisking together the ingredients. Pour over the salad, stir, and chill until required.

✳ **Serve** *with barbecued meat, lasagnes, and other family meals.*
✳ **Refrigerate** *in an airtight container for up to 24 hours.*
✳ **Variations:** *Add grated beetroot or ½ red pepper instead of the orange.*

Chicken korma

Mild kormas can contain cream, nuts, coconut or yogurt. This one uses almonds and coconut and is a delicious family meal. Curry powders and pastes are a surprisingly good source of iron.

 10 mins 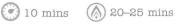 20–25 mins 1 toddler and 3 adult portions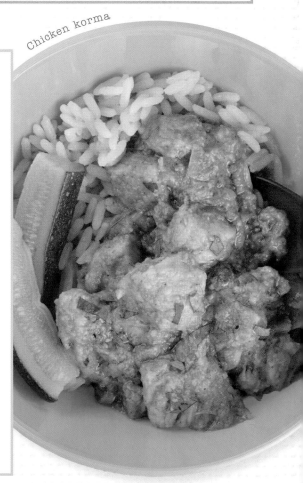

Chicken korma

ingredients

1 tbsp **vegetable oil**
1 medium **onion**, finely chopped
2 **garlic cloves**, finely chopped
400g (14oz) skinless **chicken breasts**, cut into 2cm (¾in) cubes

20g (¾oz) **korma curry powder**
50g (1¾oz) ground almonds
25g (scant 1oz) **coconut cream**, chopped or grated
1 heaped tbsp chopped **coriander**

method

1 Heat the oil in a large saucepan and gently fry the onion and garlic for 7–8 minutes, or until just softened and lightly browned. Add the chicken and cook over a low to medium heat, stirring frequently, until the chicken is just cooked on the outside.

2 Add the curry powder and mix well, cooking for about 1 minute. Stir in the almonds, 250ml (9fl oz) water, and

coconut cream, and bring the mixture to a simmering point. Stir, cover, and simmer for 10–15 minutes, or until the chicken is cooked through.

3 Sprinkle over the coriander, stir through, and remove from the heat. Allow to cool slightly before serving.

✳ **Serve** *with brown basmati rice, naan, and green vegetables or wilted spinach.*
✳ **Refrigerate** *in an airtight container for up to 24 hours.*

Chicken stir fry

To retain nutrients and keep vegetables crisp, have everything ready before you cook. Use rapeseed, sunflower or corn oil, not olive oil, which smokes with high temperatures. You can change ingredients to suit your family.

 10 mins 10 mins 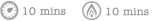 1 toddler and 3 adult portions

ingredients

2 tbsp **vegetable oil**
250g (9oz) skinless **chicken breasts**, cut into fine strips
150g (5½oz) **mangetout**, trimmed and sliced into 5mm (¼in) pieces
1 large **red** or **orange pepper**, cut into slices

200g (7oz) **beansprouts**
4 **spring onions**, trimmed and finely sliced
3cm (1in) piece of **fresh ginger** root, finely grated
2 **garlic cloves**, crushed
2 tbsp reduced-salt **soy sauce**
2 tbsp **dry sherry**

method

1 Heat 1 tablespoon of the oil in a non-stick or well-seasoned wok and, over a high heat, stir fry the chicken for 2–3 minutes, or until it is white and cooked through. Remove from the wok and keep warm.

2 Add the remaining oil and stir fry all the remaining ingredients, except the soy sauce

and sherry, for 2–3 minutes, or until they remain just crispy. If the vegetables begin to stick, add 1–2 tablespoons of water.

3 Return the chicken to the wok, stir in with the soy sauce and sherry, and serve hot with noodles or rice.

✳ *Not suitable for storing.*

✳ **Variations:** *You can use strips of pork or turkey fillet instead of chicken. Use similar quantities of finely sliced carrot or white cabbage instead of the bean sprouts or mangetout.*

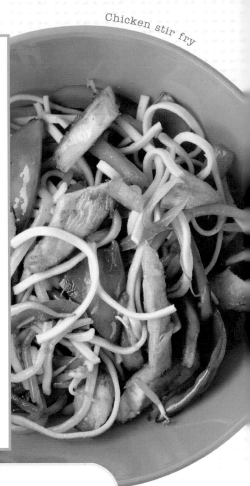

Chicken stir fry

Pork with plums

Pork loin is a lean tender cut, suitable for frying or grilling, making a succulent partner to this spicy plum sauce. Pork is particularly rich in vitamin B1.

 15 mins 20 mins 1–2 toddler and 3–4 adult portions

ingredients

1 tbsp **vegetable oil**, plus extra for brushing
2 **red onions**, finely sliced
3 **garlic cloves**, chopped
5cm (2in) **fresh ginger**, peeled and cut into fine matchsticks

1 tsp **ground mixed spice**
250g (9oz) **plums**, stoned and quartered
1 tbsp **muscovado sugar**
500g (1lb 2oz) or 2 small/1 large **pork loin** (tenderloin)

method

1 Heat the oil and sauté the onion and garlic for about 1 minute, stirring frequently.

2 Add the ginger, spice, plums, sugar, and 150ml (5fl oz) water, and allow to simmer gently for 10 minutes, or until the plums are softened. Allow to stand while you prepare the pork.

3 Preheat the oven to 150°C (300°F/Gas 2).

4 Cut the pork into 1cm (½in) slices and brush lightly with the oil. Grill in batches under a hot grill for 3–4 minutes each side, then transfer to a covered dish in the oven while you finish grilling. Serve with the plum sauce.

✳ **Serve** *with boiled rice, and steamed or stir-fried green vegetables.*

✳ *The sauce may be refrigerated for up to 24 hours or frozen when cooled. The cooked pork is not suitable for storing.*

Lamb and prune tagine

Lamb is rich in iron and zinc, and the delicious spices and succulent fruit make this a popular family meal. If you like a hot tagine, you can add a couple of dried chillies, but remove these before serving.

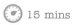 15 mins   1¾–2 hours   2 toddler and 3 adult portions

ingredients

- 2 tbsp **vegetable oil**
- 400g (14oz) lean leg or shoulder of **lamb**, cut into 2cm (¾in) cubes
- 2 medium **onions**, chopped
- 2 **garlic cloves**, crushed
- 3 tsp **ground cumin** (see tip)
- 1 tsp **ground cinnamon**
- 500ml (16fl oz) well-diluted hot **vegetable** or **lamb stock**
- 2 tbsp **tomato purée**
- 2 **lime leaves**
- 150g (5½oz) ready-to-eat **prunes**, halved, if large
- 2 tbsp chopped **coriander couscous** or **plain yogurt**, to serve (optional)

method

1 Preheat the oven to 170°C (325°F/Gas 3). Heat the oil in a non-stick pan, add the meat in batches, and stir fry until browned.

2 Add the onions and cook for a further 3 minutes, or until starting to soften. Stir in the garlic and spices and cook for a further minute, then pour in the hot stock. Stir in the purée, lime leaves, and prunes. Transfer to an ovenproof casserole, cover, and cook for 1 hour.

3 Remove from the oven, stir, and return for 30–45 minutes, or until the lamb is really tender.

4 Remove the lime leaves and stir in the coriander.

✳ **Serve** *with couscous (if you wish add parsley, lemon zest, and currants), a green leaf salad or steamed green beans.*

✳ **Refrigerate** *for up to 48 hours or freeze on the day of cooking when cool. To defrost, refrigerate overnight and reheat until piping hot.*

✳ **Tip:** *For more flavour, toast cumin seeds in a hot dry pan for a few seconds. Cool, then grind.*

Moussaka

This popular dish with aubergines, minced lamb, and an egg-enriched sauce can be varied by using beef or quorn. The aubergine in this version is lightly brushed with oil and grilled rather than fried to keep the fat content down.

 15 mins  1 hour   2 toddler and 4 adult portions

ingredients

- 1 tbsp **vegetable oil**, plus extra for greasing
- 1 large **onion**, finely chopped
- 2 **garlic cloves**, crushed
- 300g (10oz) **lean minced lamb**
- ½ tsp **ground cinnamon**
- 2 **bay leaves**
- 500ml (16fl oz) **passata**
- 2 medium **aubergines**

For the sauce:
- 25g (scant 1oz) **flour**
- 275ml (9¼fl oz) **milk**
- 10g (¼oz) **unsalted butter** or **olive spread**
- 2 **eggs**, beaten
- **black pepper**, to taste
- 20g (¾oz) **hard cheese**, such as Parmesan
- grated **nutmeg**

method

1 Preheat the oven to 200°C (400°F/Gas 6). Grease a 2-litre (3½-pint) ovenproof dish.

2 Heat some oil in a large non-stick saucepan, add the onion and garlic and fry for 5 minutes over a medium heat. Add the mince, and fry until browned, breaking up the mince with a wooden spoon.

3 Add the cinnamon, bay leaves, and passata, and bring to a simmer. Stir, cover, and simmer for 10–15 minutes. Take off the heat and remove the bay leaves.

4 Meanwhile, trim the aubergine stalks and cut lengthwise into slices roughly 1cm (½in) thick. Brush lightly with oil and place under a hot grill to soften and brown a little. Remove from the heat and allow to cool slightly.

5 Make the sauce by mixing together the flour and a little milk in a saucepan over a low heat, or jug if you prefer to make it in the microwave. When smooth, add the remaining milk and butter. Heat, stirring often, until the sauce thickens. (In the microwave, cook on high and stir every 40 seconds.) Cool a little before stirring in the eggs, pepper, and cheese.

6 Place around a third of the lamb at the base of the dish, top with half the aubergine. Repeat, finishing with the lamb. Pour the sauce over the dish and grate nutmeg on top. Bake for 25–30 minutes, or until golden brown.

✳ **Serve** *with fresh crusty bread, Wholegrain salad (see p212), steamed green vegetables or Sugar snap and apple salad (see p210).*

✳ **Refrigerate** *for up to 24 hours or freeze on the day of cooking when cooled.*

✳ **Variations:** *Lean beef or vegetarian mince, such as quorn, can be used instead of the lamb.*

Beef goulash

Goulash is a great source of iron and zinc and makes a nutritious family meal, served with noodles or mashed potatoes. Traditionally made with beef, onions, and paprika, goulash can also be made with other vegetables and spices. Paprika varies in strength; for this recipe it is best to use mild or sweet smoked paprika.

 10 mins   1¾ hours   1 toddler and 3–4 adult portions   ❄

ingredients

- 2 tbsp **vegetable oil**
- 1 medium **onion**, halved and sliced
- 2 **garlic cloves,** crushed
- 1 tbsp **plain flour** or **cornflour**
- 1–2 tsp **mild** or **sweet smoked paprika**
- 400g (14oz) **lean braising** or **casserole steak**, cut into 2cm (¾in) cubes
- 250ml (9fl oz) **water** or diluted **beef stock**
- 2 medium **green peppers**, cut into large pieces
- 400g (14oz) can chopped **tomatoes** in juice

method

1 Preheat the oven to 160°C (325°F/Gas 3).

2 Heat the oil in a large ovenproof casserole pan and fry the onion for 5 minutes, or until lightly browned. Stir in the garlic and fry for about 1 minute.

3 Coat the meat with flour by placing the flour, paprika, and meat in a clean plastic food bag and shaking. Tip the floured meat and any remaining seasoned flour into the pan and stir around briefly.

4 Add the water or stock, peppers, and tomatoes, and bring slowly to a simmering point, stirring frequently.

5 Cover and transfer to the oven and cook for 1½ hours. Check and stir, and return to the oven until the meat is really tender.

✳ **Serve** *with fat-reduced soured cream or plain yogurt, noodles, potatoes or green vegetables.*

✳ **Refrigerate** *in an airtight container for up to two days or freeze when cooled. Defrost overnight in the fridge, and, ideally, reheat in a microwave oven until piping hot before use.*

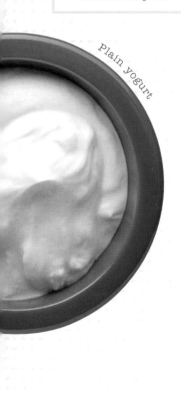

Plain yogurt

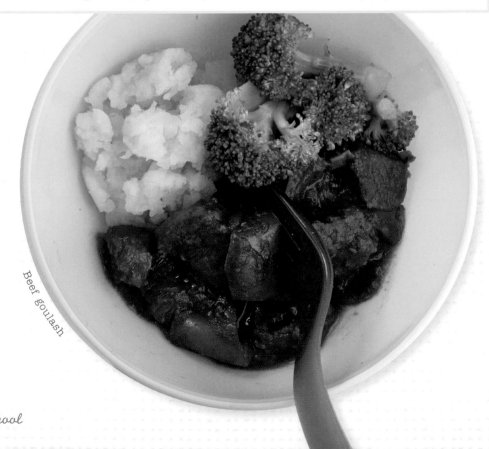

Beef goulash

Mild chilli con carne

This simple family dish can be made in bulk and frozen. It provides iron, zinc, fibre, and a host of B vitamins. Keep it mild, adding your own chilli sauce afterwards if you like.

 10 mins   40–45 mins   2 toddler and 4 adult portions ❄

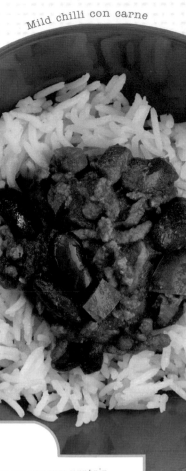

Mild chilli con carne

ingredients

2 tbsp **vegetable oil**
1 medium **onion**, finely chopped
450g (1lb) **extra lean minced beef**
1 **garlic clove**, crushed
1 large **red pepper**, deseeded and diced
½ tsp **sweet smoked paprika**
1 tsp **ground cumin**

400g (14oz) can chopped **tomatoes in juice**
2 tbsp **tomato purée**
400g (14oz) can **red kidney beans** in water, rinsed and drained
200ml (7fl oz) **water** or **beef stock**
chilli or **piri piri sauce** (optional)

method

1 Heat the oil in a large non-stick saucepan. Add the onion and cook, stirring, over a medium heat for 2–3 minutes.

2 Stir in the mince and garlic and cook for 5 minutes, or until the meat is browned, breaking up the mince with a wooden spoon. Add the remaining ingredients and bring to a simmering point.

3 Reduce the heat, cover, and cook for 30–35 minutes, stirring occasionally. Add more water if it's too thick and begins to stick to the pan.

4 When the sauce becomes thick, moist, and juicy, it is cooked. Remove your child's portion, and if you want to add some heat to your portion, add the extra chilli seasoning.

✳ **Serve** *with plain boiled rice, a baked potato or wrap in a tortilla with shredded lettuce.*

✳ **Refrigerate** *in an airtight container for up to 48 hours or freeze when cooled.*

Lasagne al forno

A succulent iron rich dish, lasagne is a worldwide classic. You can replace the meat with quorn or soya protein.

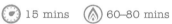 15 mins   60–80 mins   2 toddler and 4 adult portions   ❄

ingredients

For the ragu:
1 tbsp **vegetable oil**, plus extra for greasing
1 small **onion**, finely chopped
1 **garlic clove**, crushed
400g (14oz) **lean steak mince**
½ **red pepper**, finely chopped
400g (14oz) can chopped **tomatoes in juice**
2 tbsp **tomato purée**

50ml (1¾fl oz) **red wine** or **water**
2 **bay leaves**
1 tbsp chopped **thyme**

For the white sauce:
50g (1¾oz) **white flour**
500ml (16fl oz) **milk**
30g (1oz) **olive spread** or **butter**
nutmeg, to grate
150g (5½oz) **lasagne sheets**
50g (1¾oz) **Cheddar cheese**

method

1 Preheat the oven to 190°C (375°F/Gas 5). Lightly grease a lasagne dish.

2 Heat the oil in a non-stick saucepan; gently fry the onion, garlic, and mince, breaking up the meat with a wooden spoon until the mince is separated.

3 Add the pepper; fry, stirring frequently, until the vegetables are soft and the meat brown. Add the tomatoes, purée, wine or water, bay leaves, and thyme, and simmer. Stir, cover, and cook for 15–20 minutes, stirring a little. Remove the bay leaves.

4 Meanwhile, make the sauce. Whisk the flour, milk, and butter in a saucepan over a medium heat until the sauce bubbles and thickens. Cook for 1 minute. Grate in some nutmeg.

5 Pour ⅓ the ragu into the dish, add a layer of lasagne sheets, and spread a quarter of the sauce on top. Repeat until you've used up all the ragu and lasagne, then add the cheese to the remaining sauce and pour over the top. Bake for 40–45 minutes, or until the sauce is bubbling, golden brown, and the pasta soft when pierced with a sharp knife. Stand for 5 minutes then serve.

✳ **Serve** *with a salad and crusty bread.*

✳ **Refrigerate** *overnight covered in cling film or freeze in an airtight container when cooled.*

Salmon in filo pastry

Wrapping salmon in filo keeps in the moisture and looks great. This makes a handy picnic food served cold.

 5 mins 20 mins  2 toddler and 1 adult portion

ingredients

2 medium **salmon fillets**, preferably skinless
4–5 filo **pastry sheets**
juice of ½ **lemon** or **lime**
1 tbsp chopped **parsley**
vegetable oil, for brushing

method

1 Preheat the oven to 200°C (400°F/Gas 6).

2 Remove the salmon's skin, if not skinned already, and check for bones by running your finger over the flesh; remove any you find. Cut off a thumb-sized piece for your baby's portion.

3 Lay a sheet of filo pastry on a clean surface; spray or brush with oil. Place 1 baby piece of salmon near the short end of the pastry rectangle, squeeze over lemon, and add a little parsley. Roll the pastry over to cover the fish, and tuck in the sides. Once you have a little parcel, put this on a lightly oiled baking sheet and spray or brush with oil.

4 Make 2 baby portions, then repeat for the adult portion. If the salmon is visible, use 1 more sheet, oiling first so it sticks. Bake for 20 minutes, or until golden brown. Cool a little before serving.

＊**Serve** *hot with mixed vegetables, new potatoes or salad.*

＊**Refrigerate** *in an airtight container for up to 24 hours.*

＊**Variations:** *Add chopped spring onions, and/or slices of red pepper, or asparagus pieces in season.*

Tuna pasta bake

Each family has its own version of this dish, which is a meal in itself. It's a great standby as most of the ingredients are storecupboard basics.

 20 mins 15–30 mins 2 toddler and 3 adult portions

ingredients

250g (9oz) **penne pasta**
vegetable oil (optional)
100g (3½oz) **peas**, defrosted
100g (3½oz) **sweetcorn kernels**, frozen defrosted, or canned in water
2 x 185g (6½oz) cans of **tuna** in water, drained

For the sauce:
500ml (16fl oz) **whole milk**
50g (1¼oz) **flour**
30g (1oz) **butter** or **olive spread**
1 tsp ready-made **mustard** (optional)
2 tbsp **tomato purée**
50g (1¾oz) **Cheddar cheese**

method

1 Cook the pasta in boiling water until just tender, and drain. Return to the saucepan, cover, and add a dribble of oil, if needed, to prevent from sticking to the pan.

2 Meanwhile, make the sauce by placing the milk, flour, and butter in a large saucepan and whisking over a medium heat until it bubbles and thickens. Reduce the heat and cook for 2 minutes. Stir in the mustard, if using, tomato purée, and half the cheese.

3 Add the peas, sweetcorn, tuna, and pasta, and stir well. Pour into a flameproof dish, sprinkle over the remaining cheese, and put under a preheated grill for 4–5 minutes, or until the cheese bubbles and browns. Or place in a preheated oven at 180°C (350°F/Gas 4) and bake for 15–20 minutes. Cool for 1–2 minutes before serving.

＊**Serve** *with additional green vegetables or a side salad.*

＊**Refrigerate** *for 24 hours. Reheat until piping hot, preferably in a microwave to prevent it from drying out.*

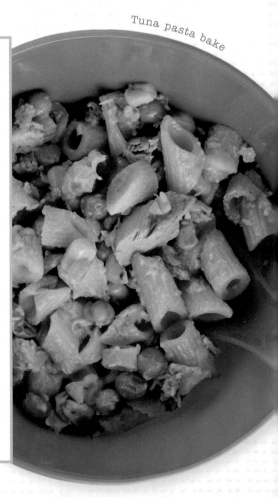

Tuna pasta bake

Vegetarian lasagne

These come in many forms, some using lentils or beans, others soya mince or quorn. This uses a type of vitamin-C rich ratatouille that makes a delicious moist lasagne.

 20 mins  70–75 mins 2 toddler and 4 adult portions

ingredients

2 tbsp **olive oil**, plus extra for greasing
1 medium **onion**, sliced
2 **garlic cloves**, chopped
1 medium **red** or **yellow pepper**, cut into chunks
1 medium **aubergine**, cut into 1cm (½in) cubes

1 **courgette** sliced
2 x 400g (14oz) can chopped **tomatoes in juice**
1 tbsp **mixed chopped herbs**, such as oregano/thyme
150g (5½oz) **lasagne verdi sheets**

For the sauce:
50g (1¾oz) **plain flour**
500ml (16fl oz) **milk**
30g (1oz) **unsalted butter** or **olive spread**
grated nutmeg
75g (2½oz) strong **Cheddar cheese**, grated

method

1 Preheat the oven to 190°C (375°F/Gas 5). Lightly grease a large lasagne dish.

2 Heat the oil in a saucepan. Fry the onion and garlic for 5 minutes, or until just soft. Add the pepper; fry for 2–3 minutes.

3 Stir in the aubergine, courgette, tomatoes, and herbs. Bring the mixture to a simmering point, stir, and cover. Cook for 20 minutes while you make the sauce, stirring occasionally.

4 Whisk the flour and milk in a saucepan, and add the butter. Heat, whisking continuously, until the sauce bubbles and thickens. Cook for 1 minute, and grate in some nutmeg.

5 Pour or spoon around a third of the mixture into the dish, add a layer of lasagne sheets, and spread a quarter of the sauce on top. Repeat until you've used all the vegetables and lasagne, add the cheese to the rest of the sauce, and pour over the top.

6 Bake for 40–45 minutes, or until the sauce is bubbling, golden, and the pasta soft when pierced with a sharp knife. Stand for 5 minutes before serving.

* **Serve** *with a green salad, Wholegrain salad (see p212) or crusty bread.*

* **Refrigerate** *in an airtight container for up to 24 hours or freeze when cooled.*

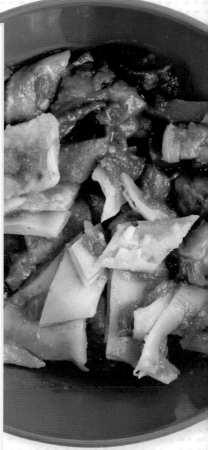

Vegetarian lasagne

Vegetable chow mein

A delicious and speedy meal that is full of nutritious vegetables, topped with crunchy cashew nuts.

 5 mins 10 mins 1 toddler and 2 adult portions

ingredients

250g (9oz) **egg noodles**
1 tbsp **sesame** or **vegetable oil**
2 tbsp **vegetable oil**
2 **garlic cloves**, chopped
3cm (1in) piece **fresh ginger**, finely grated
100g (3½oz) **mushrooms**, sliced
1 **red** or **orange pepper**, finely sliced
2 tbsp **dry sherry**

2 tbsp low-salt **soy sauce**
1 head **pak choi**, sliced
100g (3½oz) **beansprouts**, rinsed and well drained
4 **spring onions**, in 1cm (½in) slices
100g (3½oz) **cashew nuts**, toasted
1 tbsp chopped **coriander** (optional)

method

1 Cook the noodles according to the packet instructions. Rinse, drain, and toss in the sesame oil to separate them. Put to one side while you cook the stir fry.

2 Heat the oil in a wok. Add the garlic and ginger, frying briefly, then the mushrooms and pepper. Stir fry for 2–3 minutes. Add the sherry and soy sauce, quickly followed by the noodles, pak choi, beansprouts, and spring onions, stirring continuously. Add 1 tablespoon of water if sticky.

3 Serve with sprinkled cashews, and coriander, if using.

* *Not suitable for storage.*

* **Variations:** *Omit or replace the cashews with plain unsalted toasted peanuts.*

Dealing with choking

As a new parent it is a good idea to attend a special baby and child first aid course with one of the first aid training organisations so that you know what to do if an emergency affects a child in your care. These courses will teach you everything from how to treat cuts and choking to what to do if your child ever loses consciousness. You will learn how to give cardiopulmonary resuscitation (CPR), a combination of chest compressions and rescue breaths, which is a potentially life-saving technique used to treat a child who has stopped breathing.

How to deal with choking

A baby can choke on small pieces of food or after putting a small object in his or her mouth. Don't intervene if your baby is able to cough as your action could cause the obstruction to move further down the airway, but if he or she becomes distressed and is unable to breathe or make a noise treat as described below.

- If your baby is distressed, is unable to cry, cough or breathe, you need to take emergency action to clear her airway. Lay her face down along your thigh and support her head and upper body with one hand. Using the heel of your other hand, give up to five sharp blows to the upper part of her back between the shoulder blades.

- Turn her over so that she is face up along your other leg and check her mouth. If you can clearly see a loose object, remove it carefully with your fingertips. Do not sweep the inside of her mouth with your fingers or feel blindly down her throat as you may push an object further in or damage her throat.

- If the back blows have not cleared the obstruction, try chest thrusts. With the baby lying face up along your leg, support her upper body and head with one hand and give up to five chest thrusts, by pushing down with two fingers of your other hand on the lower part of the breastbone.

- Check quickly after each chest thrust to see if the obstruction has been dislodged. If the obstruction does not clear after three cycles of five back blows and five chest thrusts, call for an ambulance.

- Continue giving cycles of back blows then mouth checks, and chest thrusts then mouth checks until the ambulance arrives.

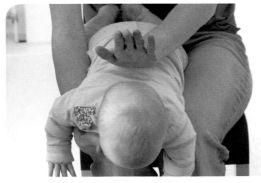

Giving back blows
Make sure the baby's head is lower than her body. Keeping your fingers raised, use the heel of your hand to give back blows; make sure the blows fall between her shoulder blades.

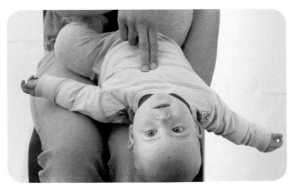

Giving chest thrusts
Place your first two fingers on the lower half of the baby's breastbone; make sure they are not on the ribs. Push inwards and downwards towards the baby's head.

Index

Useful resources

www.nhs.uk/conditions/pregnancy-and-baby/pages/
solid-foods-weaning.aspx
Advice on weaning babies

www.infantandtoddlerforum.org
Expert advice for professionals and families on feeding
preschool children

www.childrensfoodtrust.org.uk
Government-backed website providing information for early
years carers on healthy eating for young children

www.healthystart.nhs.uk
Information on healthy living for young children

www.cwt.org.uk
Charity that aims to improve public health through healthy
eating

www.nutrition.org.uk/healthyliving/nutrition4baby
British Nutrition Foundation information on maternal and
infant nutrition

www.bda.uk.com/foodfacts/index.html#babies
Professional website for UK dietitians

www.babycentre.co.uk
Information and advice on caring for babies and young
children

www.vegsoc.org
Vegetarian society website with information on vegetarian
diets for children

www.rapleyweaning.com
Information and advice on following baby-led weaning

www.allergyuk.org
Charity website with information and advice on weaning
and food allergies in young children

www.tommys.org
Website for parents with premature babies

www.tamba.org.uk
Website for parents with twins

First Aid societies
www.redcross.org.uk
www.sja.org.uk
www.firstaid.org.uk

Acknowledgments

Author's acknowledgments

Thank you Dorling Kindersley for giving me the
opportunity to write a book that combines both my
experience in infant nutrition and creativity in the kitchen.
I hope that for readers it provides an authoritative guide
to feeding in the early years, giving practical advice,
delicious nutritious recipes, and clear information.

I'd like to acknowledge the team I've worked with on
this book, whose enthusiasm and commitment has been
exemplary. So thank you Claire for being a great editor,
and Harriet for bringing the pages to life with your
beautiful images and creativity. Thank you too to Anna
for her "big picture" perspective, and Lizzie for her
efficiency behind the scenes.

Thanks also are due to my family whose meals have been
somewhat unusual whilst the recipes progressed, but who
at least were spared stage one recipes!

Publisher's acknowledgments

DK would like to thank Claire Wedderburn-Maxwell for
proofreading; Marie Lorimer for the index; Liz Hippisley
for prop styling; Georgie Besterman for food styling; Dr
Su Laurent for consulting on the premature baby spread;
and Dr Carol Cooper for consulting on the allergy spread.
Thanks to Collette Sadler for design assistance and
Elizabeth Clinton for editorial assistance.

All images © Dorling Kindersley. For more information
see www.dkimages.com